FOOD FOR RUGBY

Eat Well, Perform Better

FOOD FOR RUGBY

Eat Well, Perform Better

Jane Griffin

With a Foreword by Keith Wood

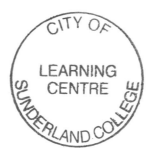

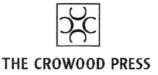

THE CROWOOD PRESS

First published in 2007 by
The Crowood Press Ltd
Ramsbury, Marlborough
Wiltshire SN8 2HR

www.crowood.com

British Library Cataloguing-in-Publication Data
A catalogue record for this book is available from the British Library.

ISBN 978 1 86126 695 8

Disclaimer
Please note that the author and the publisher of this book do not accept
any responsibility whatsoever for any error or omission, nor any loss,
injury, damage, adverse outcome or liability suffered as a result of the
information contained in this book, or reliance upon it. Playing rugby
could involve physical activities that are too strenuous for some individuals
to engage in safely, and before making dietary changes and/or engaging in
rugby training a doctor should be consulted.

Typeset by Carolyn Griffiths

Printed and bound in India by Replika Press

CONTENTS

Foreword

I first met Jane Griffin when the professional game was introduced in 1996. Professionalism was not just about getting paid to play, but was also the changing of ideas in order to bring the game to the heights of the players' ability. In the amateur days we all worked and rugby was very much a hobby, although one of huge personal importance; however, our ambition never reached fulfilment because we never prepared properly. Our training and lifestyle was of a low standard, and it took us a long time to raise the bar. Jane was instrumental in my own journey from over-weight fatty to captain of my country; there was no quick fix, just a re-education of my dietary life to maximize my performance. At times it was very tough, and even now I look back and wish I had taken a far better view to nutrition in my teens. I was late in learning, but Jane's intervention meant I had a lot of years at the top. In order to train properly and to play at a high level, nutrition is vitally important: Jane's common-sense approach is ideal for the professional rugby player.

Keith Wood

Introduction

What players eat and drink can help them to achieve their performance goals, remain healthy and to a certain extent avoid injury. Given the nature of the sport and the amount of contact that takes place in both training and matches, obviously not all injuries can be avoided – but diet can certainly help in the recovery process. The energy demands of training and matches can increase daily requirements by up to 1,000kcal a day. However, this is not an excuse to eat anything as long as it supplies the energy. The body can only store a given amount of carbohydrate in the muscles, unlike fat which can be stored in unlimited amounts. Yet it is carbohydrate that is the key fuel for rugby players, and poor stores can lead to early fatigue in training sessions and matches and an increased risk of injury as the muscle begins to tire. Many years ago, the advice was basically just to increase intake. Now players must consider not just how much to eat, but what type of carbohydrate-rich food or drink is best before, during and immediately after exercise.

Unlike many team sports, there are more opportunities to take fluids on board during matches. However, many players are not aware of the importance of keeping hydrated, and of the negative effects that dehydration can have on both physical and mental performance. As players become dehydrated they start to fatigue not only physically, but mentally too: errors start to creep in as concentration dips, reaction times slow up, and decision making, anticipation and skill delivery all slump. The hydration status of two players from opposing teams could be the difference between a match-winning try and a try-saving tackle.

Brought up in Manchester, my older brother and my father would take me to see Sale when they were playing at home. In those days backs and forwards were easily identifiable. Though I had no idea at that age that I would one day be a sports dietitian, my untrained eye could tell that some players were – and there is no polite way to say this – fatter than others. Nowadays players are all lean, regardless of their position. As a result, Chapter 5 has been devoted to 'gaining muscle' and Chapter 6 to 'losing body fat'. Often the requirement for a player is to do both, which may seem to some like an impossible task. Surely you eat less to lose body fat, and eat more to gain muscle? Find out if this is true by turning to these chapters.

Having been involved as a sports dietitian in rugby for over twelve years, perhaps the most irritating aspect of the game (and it is not just rugby that this annoyance applies to) is the belief that supplements are the answer to everything. Some do have a role to play: a dietary supplement may temporarily plug a nutritional gap while a player works hard to improve his or her diet. Creatine supplementation has been scientifically proven to aid performance, particularly during intensive strength training. However, there are many supplements that have not been proven to help in any way: some have led to positive drug tests, others have been expensive purchases but without any obvious benefits. Supplements are just that: supplements to the diet, not short-cuts. With few exceptions, improving the diet will have the biggest impact on performance.

Young players have enormous energy and nutrient requirements, as these must meet the demands of growth and development as well as their sport. For many this is an uphill struggle, particularly when access to food at school and college may be limited in quality as well as quantity. Young players not only need advice about what, when and how much to eat and drink, they invariably need practical advice about shopping and cooking. One last group of players who could benefit from sound advice about diet are those players unlucky enough to get injured. Broken jaws obviously require special dietary advice, but a sudden change in activity level can lead to problems of weight gain (as body fat) if sensible dietary adjustments are not made.

From my years of working with rugby players, I have found it is important to explain why dietary changes need to be made, and the positive effects these changes could have on performance in training and matches. This can then be followed by sound, practical advice to help bring about these changes. I hope this is what I have achieved with this book, and that you will find the 'whys' and the 'hows' informative and helpful, and that you enjoy reading and using *Food for Rugby*.

Jane Griffin
Sports Dietitian and Nutrition Consultant

Acknowledgements

To my husband Chris for his love, support, encouragement and sound advice. To my children Daniel and Jessica for their love and particularly their awareness that a closed study door means 'do not disturb'! To my brother Robin for more sound advice, and who with my late father took me to watch Sale play when I was a little girl.

To all the players I have worked with and learnt so much from, and particularly all the England Rugby Academy players at London Irish, NEC Harlequins and London Wasps who make my job such fun.

CHAPTER 1

The Basics

Players rely on what they eat and drink on a daily basis to supply all their energy needs and nutrient requirements. The only exception is vitamin D, which is made by the action of sunlight on the skin; this makes dietary requirement very small, or even unnecessary, particularly when one considers how much time a player will spend outside training and playing matches. If the food choices and amounts eaten each day do not meet these requirements, performance will suffer, the risk of infections will increase, injuries may take longer to mend, and there could even be long-term health implications, too.

Not only do nutrients have different functions in the body, but the type and amount of nutrients vary from food to food. Understanding what energy and nutrients do in the body, and which foods are good sources of particular nutrients, will help a player build up the best possible diet in order to maximize his performance in training and matches, and keep the body fit and healthy. The diet must be practical, it must fit into a player's lifestyle and daily schedule, and of course it must be enjoyable.

NUTRIENTS AND THEIR MAIN FUNCTIONS

Food is made up of carbohydrate, fat, protein, vitamins, minerals and water. In some foods, particularly fruits and vegetables, a very large proportion is water; in others, such as oils and fats, the water content is minimal. The amounts, and indeed the presence of the different vitamins and minerals, can vary considerably between foods, too. This is why health professionals, including sports dietitians and registered sports nutritionists, are constantly encouraging people to eat a diet that contains a wide variety of different foods.

Carbohydrate and fat are the major sources of energy or fuel for the body. Protein has the unique function of providing the material for growth and repair of the body. Vitamins and minerals are essential nutrients, which must be supplied by the diet, and although the majority of them are needed in very small amounts, they do play vital and different roles in the diet. Vitamins are a diverse group of substances that are needed for the regulation of chemical processes in the body. Though not a source of energy themselves, many of them are involved in the release of energy from food. Minerals such as vitamins also fulfil many functions: they help to control the composition of body fluids, they are constituents of bones and teeth, and are essential components of enzymes and proteins such as haemoglobin.

How Much is Enough?

In 1991 the United Kingdom Department of Health published revised guidelines for the intake of nutrients using the term Reference Nutrient Intake (*see* References Chapter 1, 1). This was defined as the amount of a nutrient that is enough for almost every individual, even someone who has high needs for it. It is therefore considerably higher than most people need, and as long as individuals are consuming the RNI of a nutrient, they are most unlikely to be deficient in that nutrient.

Energy

All the energy needed by the body comes from the diet. Food is digested, absorbed and metabolized to release energy that the body can use.

The Energy Value of Food		
1g protein	→	4kcals
1g fat	→	9kcals
1g carbohydrate	→	3.75kcals
1g alcohol	→	7kcals
1g water	→	0kcals

Almost all the weight of food is made up of these components plus water. Therefore foods that contain a large percentage of water, such as fruits and vegetables, will have relatively fewer calories, and fatty foods that contain little water, such as butter, margarines and oils, will be rich in calories. In fact most foods are a mixture of nutrients, and the total energy value of a food is therefore the sum of the energy from each of the nutrients.

THE CONSTITUENTS OF FOOD

Carbohydrate

Carbohydrate occurs in the diet as simple carbohydrate or sugar, and complex carbohydrate or starch. Most dietary carbohydrate is

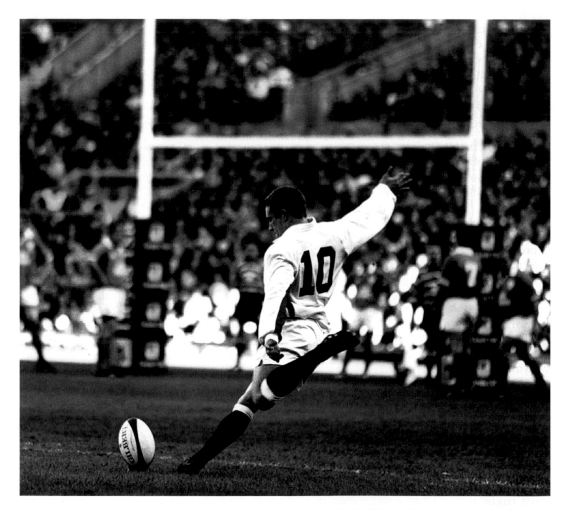

England's Johnny Wilkinson takes a kick at goal in the England v. Ireland game in the Lloyd's TSB Six Nations Championship game at Twickenham in 2002. (© PA Photos)

plant in origin apart from lactose, the sugar that is found in milk. The main sources of simple carbohydrates are fruits and fruit juices, milk and milk products, honey and sugar. Contrary to popular belief, sugar occurs naturally as sugarcane and sugar beet, and in lesser amounts in fruits and some root vegetables such as carrots. Sugar, or more correctly termed sucrose, is made up of a combination of two other simple sugars: glucose and fructose. Sugar, whether it is brown or white, is pure sucrose. All these foods are identifiable by their sweet taste. Sources of complex carbohydrates include bread, rice, potatoes, breakfast cereals, pulses and sweetcorn.

Carbohydrates are the most important source of energy in the diet, being vital sources for exercising muscles, the brain and the central nervous system. People who try to follow currently fashionable low carbohydrate/high protein diets soon begin to realize the role that carbohydrates play in the body because they feel tired, lethargic and irritable as the body becomes deprived of stored carbohydrate. Unfortunately the body can only store carbohydrate in limited amounts in the liver and muscles as glycogen.

Dietary Fibre

Fibre – originally called roughage – is now referred to as 'non-starch polysaccharide' (NSP). However, even though the latter is technically correct, dietary fibre is still the term most people use, and remains the term used in food labelling.

Fibre is the major component of plant cell walls; it is resistant to the action of digestive enzymes. Most dietary fibre comes from fruit, vegetables and cereals, and it can be soluble or insoluble. Insoluble fibre helps to keep the bowels functioning healthily and regularly; it swells in the gut as it absorbs water, making the gut contents heavier, resulting in a quicker movement through the digestive system. This can help to relieve constipation (not a common complaint among most rugby players) and other bowel disorders. The fibre is mainly insoluble in wheat, maize and rice.

Soluble fibre occurs more in oats, legumes, leafy vegetables and some fruits, particularly apples. It is thought to help reduce blood cholesterol levels and slow down the absorption of blood glucose in some types of diabetes. As a result the general population is being encouraged to increase their intake of dietary fibre. Players who include plenty of carbohydrate in their diet for other reasons will certainly meet their requirement for dietary fibre without including any particularly high fibre foods.

Fat

Fat is an essential nutrient and an important source of energy, and although many people consume excessive amounts it should not be excluded from the diet, only limited in some cases. Fat also supplies the essential fatty acids, the omega-3 and omega-6 families. The body cannot manufacture these fatty acids and therefore must rely on dietary supplies. Fat provides insulation and cushioning for the internal organs, and it also serves as a carrier for the fat-soluble vitamins and antioxidants. Some fats are vital for the formation of hormones.

Many of the flavours, smells and textures of food are linked to the fats in it: without some fat in the diet, food would taste bland. However, an excessive amount of fat in the diet has become increasingly recognized as one of the risk factors influencing the development of chronic diseases. The main concern is centred on the part that high intakes of fat play in contributing to obesity and all its associated health risks such as heart disease. The presence of fat in some foods is very obvious (visible fat), but less obvious in others (invisible fat). If a player needs to reduce their fat intake as part of a programme to reduce body fat content, controlling the intake of the foods with large amounts of invisible fat will obviously be much more of a challenge. In this situation a player should concentrate on cutting out foods that contribute few nutrients (fast foods and pastry) but continue to include foods with an all-round nutritional value (cheese and eggs).

Sources of Fat

Visible fat	Invisible fat
Butter, margarine	Very lean cuts of meat
Oils, lard, suet, dripping	Cheese
Hydrogenated fats and vegetable shortening	Whole milk
(check food labels)	Eggs
Cream	Meat products: pies, pasties,
Fat on meat, poultry skin	sausages, burgers, pâté, salami, tinned meats
Oily fish	Chips, crisps and roast potatoes
	Fried food and pastry
	Nuts, olives, avocado pears
	Some cakes and biscuits
	Creamy puddings and cheesecake
	Mayonnaise, salad cream, creamy sauces
	Peanut butter
	Chocolate, toffee, fudge

Protein

Protein performs vital structural functions in the body and is found in muscle, bone, cartilage, tendons, ligaments, skin and hair. The body needs protein for growth and development, and it is constantly involved in rebuilding, repairing and maintaining vital tissues. Enzymes are proteins acting as catalysts, regulating and accelerating the rate of biochemical reactions taking place in the body. Some hormones are also proteinous in nature, including insulin, which is responsible for preventing excessive levels of glucose accumulating in the blood by enabling its uptake by cells.

Other proteins are important in the functioning of the immune system, and have roles to play in fighting off infections. Yet others work as transporters, moving fats and minerals around the body: for example, oxygen is transported in the blood to all cells by the protein haemoglobin. Although these are the primary and unique functions of protein, it can be used as a source of energy, too. However, unlike fat and to a lesser extent carbohydrate, it cannot be stored in the body. If more protein is eaten than the body needs, part of the protein molecule is broken down and excreted in the urine as urea, and the remainder is used either as an immediate energy source or it is converted to fat and stored.

Sources of Protein

Animal sources	Vegetable sources
Meat	Beans, peas and
Offal (kidney, liver etc.)	lentils
Poultry	Nuts and seeds
Fish (white, oily	Quorn and tofu
and shellfish)	Soya beans, soya
Eggs	milk
Milk, cheese, yogurt	Textured vegetable
	protein
	Bread, potatoes,
	rice, pasta, cereals

Amino Acids

Amino acids are the building blocks of protein. All the proteins needed by the body can be made from just twenty different amino acids: some can be made from others and are called non-essential amino acids, but there are others that cannot be made by the body and have to be supplied by the diet – these are known as essential amino acids. Cysteine and tyrosine are sometimes called semi-essential amino acids as they can only be made from the essential amino acids methionine and phenylalanine.

Classification of Amino Acids	
Essential amino acids	**Non-essential amino acids**
Isoleucine	Alanine
Leucine	Arginine
Lysine	Asparagine
Methionine	Aspartic acid
Phenylalanine	Cysteine/cystine
Threonine	Glutamic acid
Tryptophan	Glutamine
Valine	Glycine
Histidine (in infants)	Proline
	Serine
	Tyrosine

Animal or Vegetable?

Some foods contain more protein than others, but actually quality is just as important as quantity: it is not merely the amount of protein that matters, but also which amino acids the protein contains, and whether they are present in sufficient amounts. Thus:

- Plant proteins tend to be low or even deficient in one or more essential amino acids and therefore generally have a lower biological value than animal proteins.
- Animal foods – for example meat, fish, eggs, milk and cheese – have a high protein content with a high biological value.
- Pulses – for example soya bean, kidney beans, chickpeas, lentils and peanuts – are foods with a very high protein content, with a high (soya) or medium biological value.
- Cereals – wheat, rice, barley, maize and oats – have a medium protein content and low biological value, with the exception of rice, which has a medium biological value.
- Nuts – hazelnut, cashew, almond, walnut – have a high protein content but a low biological value.
- Starchy roots (cassava, potato, yam and sweet potato) are low in protein and have a negligible biological value.
- Vegetables and fruits are low in protein and are not really considered dietary sources of protein, though of course they make a valuable contribution to the diet in many other ways.

Too Much Protein in the Diet

A high protein diet increases the workload of the kidneys because of the extra nitrogen that must be excreted. This does not seem to be a problem in otherwise healthy people, but it might be in physically active individuals who already have increased fluid losses through sweating.

Vitamins

Vitamins are complex organic substances needed in very small but vital amounts in the body. The diet must provide them all as they cannot be made by the body, with the one exception of vitamin D.

Vitamins have a variety of functions in the body. Some are co-factors in enzyme activity, some are antioxidants and vitamin D is a pro-hormone. Vitamin deficiency diseases are rare in the UK, though they still occur in some parts of the world. Vitamins are either fat soluble and stored in the body (vitamins A, D, E and K), or water soluble and not stored in the body (vitamin C and the B-complex vitamins). Any water-soluble vitamins consumed in excess of requirements will normally be excreted via the kidneys in the urine.

Vitamin A

Major food sources:

- Vitamin A is found in animal foods as retinol. Plant foods contain beta-carotene, the precursor of vitamin A.
- The richest sources of vitamin A are fish liver oils (cod liver oil) and animal liver (lamb, calf and pig).
- Good sources of vitamin A include oily fish (mackerel, herring, tuna, sardines and salmon), egg yolk, full fat milk, butter, cheese and fortified margarine.
- Good sources of beta-carotene are fruit and vegetables, especially orange ones (carrots, apricots), dark green ones (spinach, watercress and broccoli) and red ones (tomatoes and red peppers).

Main functions:

- Essential for healthy skin.
- Maintains healthy mucous membranes in the throat and nose.

- Protects against poor vision in dim light.
- Antioxidant properties.

Deficiency: Very rare in this country. In Third World countries deficiency is a major cause of blindness.

Requirement: Reference Nutrient Intake (RNI) for adult women is 600µg per day, and for adult men 700µg per day.

Excessive intakes: Regular intakes of retinol should not exceed 7,500µg for adult women, 9,000µg for adult men and 3,300µg for pregnant women. Women who are, or who might become pregnant are advised by the Department of Health not to take vitamin A supplements or to eat liver, as excessive amounts can be toxic and dangerous to the unborn child.

Vitamin B1 (Thiamin)
Major food sources: Cereal products such as breakfast cereals, bread, pasta and rice, lean pork and peas, beans and lentils.

Main functions: The release of energy from carbohydrate, and for the normal functioning of nerves, brain and muscles.

Deficiency: Very rare in this country. Causes beri-beri, which affects the heart and nervous system.

Requirements: RNI 1.0mg per day for adult men, and 0.8mg per day for adult women. (Dependent on the energy content of the diet, an RNI is set at 0.4mg per 1,000kcals for most groups of people.)

Excessive intakes: Chronic intakes in excess of 3g per day are toxic in adults.

Vitamin B2 (Riboflavin)
Major food sources: Milk, egg yolks, liver, kidneys, cheese, wholemeal bread and cereals and green vegetables. Sensitive to light.

Main functions: The release of energy from carbohydrate, fat and protein.

Deficiency: Sores in the corners of the mouth. Severe deficiency is unlikely in the UK.

Requirements: RNI for adult men is 1.3mg per day, and for adult women 1.1mg per day.

Excessive intakes: The absorption of riboflavin in the intestine is limited, so toxic effects are unlikely.

Niacin (Nicotinic Acid, Nicotinamide, Vitamin B3)
Major food sources: Meat, poultry, fortified breakfast cereals, white flour and bread, yeast extracts.

Main functions: The release of energy from protein, fat and carbohydrate.

Deficiency: Rare.

Requirements: RNI for adult men is 17mg per day, and for adult women 13mg per day.

Excessive intakes: Very high intakes in the region of 3–6g per day may cause liver damage.

Vitamin B6 (Pyridoxine)
Major food sources: Meat, particularly beef and poultry, fish, wholemeal bread and fortified breakfast cereals.

Main functions: Needed for protein metabolism, the function of the central nervous system, haemoglobin production and antibody formation.

Deficiency: Deficiency signs are rare.

Requirements: RNI for adult men is 1.4mg per day, and for adult women 1.2mg per day.

Excessive intakes: High intakes have been associated with impaired function of the sensory nerves. Amounts involved have varied from 50mg per day, to 2 to 7g per day.

Vitamin B12 (Cyanocobalamin)
Major food sources: Found only in food of animal origin (liver, kidney, meat, oily fish,

milk, cheese and eggs). Some breakfast cereals are fortified with vitamin B12. Some vegetarian foods are fortified, for example soya protein, soya milks, yeast extract.

Main functions: Red blood-cell formation, maintenance of the nervous system, and protein metabolism.

Deficiency: Pernicious anaemia (blood disorder).

Requirement: The RNI for adult men and women is 1.5µg per day.

Excessive intakes: Excreted in the urine and therefore not dangerous.

Folic Acid (Folates)
Major food sources: Liver, kidney, green leafy vegetables, wholegrain cereals, fortified breakfast cereals and breads, eggs, pulses, bananas and orange juice.

Main functions: Red and white blood cell formation in bone marrow. Essential for growth. Protection against neural tube defects (spina bifida) pre-conceptually and in early pregnancy.

Deficiency: Megaloblastic anaemia (blood disorder).

Requirement: RNI for adults is 200µg per day. Women who might become pregnant, or pregnant women during the first twelve weeks of pregnancy, are recommended to take an extra 400µg per day.

Excessive intakes: Dangers of toxicity are very low.

Biotin and Pantothenic Acid
Major food sources: Widespread in food.

Main functions: Release of energy from fats, carbohydrates and protein.

Deficiency: Unlikely.

Requirement: None set.

Excessive intakes: No danger.

Vitamin C
Major food sources: Fruit and vegetables, especially blackcurrants, strawberries and citrus fruit, raw peppers, tomatoes and green leafy vegetables; potatoes because of the amount eaten.

Main functions: For healthy skin, blood vessels, gums and teeth, wound healing, iron absorption and formation of antibodies. It is an important antioxidant.

Deficiency: Will cause scurvy. A mild deficiency leads to tiredness, bleeding gums, delayed wound healing and lowered resistance to infection.

Requirement: RNI for adults is 40mg per day.

Excessive intakes: Intakes at levels of twenty times the RNI or more have been associated with diarrhoea and the increased risk of oxalate stones in the kidney.

Vitamin D (Cholecalciferol)
Major food sources: Fortified margarines and spreads, fortified breakfast cereals, oily fish, egg yolks, full fat milk and dairy products. The main source of vitamin D is the action of UV light on the skin.

Main function: The absorption of calcium and its utilization in the body, particularly the mineralization of bones and teeth.

Deficiency: Loss of calcium from the bones, causing rickets in young children and osteomalacia, particularly in women of child-bearing age.

Requirement: No dietary source is needed for adults, provided that the skin is exposed to sunlight (the RNI for adults aged sixty-five and over is 10µg per day).

Excessive intakes: Toxicity is rare in adults.

Vitamin E
Major food sources: Vegetable oils, seeds, nuts (especially peanuts), wheatgerm, wholemeal bread and cereals, green plants, milk and milk products and egg yolks.

Main functions: Powerful antioxidant, protecting body tissues against free radical damage.

Deficiency: None, except in very exceptional circumstances.

Requirement: No RNI set: 4mg per day for adult men and 3mg per day for adult women is considered adequate.

Excessive intakes: Toxicity is extremely rare.

Vitamin K
Major food sources: Dark green leafy vegetables, margarines and vegetable oils, milk and liver. Also synthesized by bacteria in the gut.

Main functions: Blood clotting.

Deficiency: Rare in adults.

Requirement: No RNI is set, but 1μg per kg per day is considered both safe and adequate.

Excessive intakes: Natural K vitamins seem free from toxic side effects, even up to a hundred times the safe intake. Synthetic forms may not have such a margin of safety.

Minerals

Minerals are inorganic substances needed by the body for a wide range of vital functions. They are involved in building and maintaining strong bones and teeth, transporting oxygen around the body, regulating water and acid–base balance, activating and forming essential parts of enzymes and hormones, fighting infections, maintaining healthy levels of haemoglobin in the blood, releasing energy from food, transmitting nerve impulses and relaxing and contracting muscles. Most minerals need to be supplied on a regular basis by the diet. While deficiencies in essential nutrients can be harmful, so can excessive amounts too. Both must be avoided.

Calcium
Major food sources: Milk, cheese and yogurt (low fat and full fat), tinned sardines and pilchards (from the edible bones), dark green leafy vegetables, pulses (including baked beans), white flour and white bread (fortified) and hard water.

Main functions: Essential for strong and healthy bones and teeth. Important in blood clotting. Essential for nerve and muscle function.

Deficiency: Causes problems with bones, which may become brittle and break easily (osteoporosis or brittle bone disease). Good calcium intakes in childhood and adolescence are vital to help build up calcium in the bones and to protect against osteoporosis in later life.

Requirement: RNI for adult men and women is 700mg per day. Vitamin D is essential for the absorption of calcium.

Excessive intakes: Calcium toxicity is virtually unknown. The body adapts to high intakes by reducing the amount that is absorbed.

Phosphorus
Major food sources: Present in all plant and animal foods except fats and sugars.

Main functions: Essential for the formation of bones and teeth. Involved in many metabolic reactions.

Deficiency: Unknown.

Requirement: RNI for adult men and women is 550mg per day.

Excessive intakes: Not known in adults.

Magnesium
Major food sources: Present in most foods, particularly cereals, vegetables (especially dark green leafy ones) and fruit.

Main functions: Energy production, nerve and muscle function and bone structure.

Deficiency: Body is very efficient at regulating magnesium content so deficiencies are rare. Usually caused by severe diarrhoea or excessive losses in the urine resulting from the use of diuretics.

Requirements: The RNI for adult men is 300mg per day and for adult women 270mg per day.

Excessive intakes: There is no evidence that high intakes are harmful if kidney function is normal.

Sodium and Chloride

Major food sources: As sodium chloride (salt). About 15–20 per cent sodium chloride in the diet is naturally present in food, 15–29 per cent is added in cooking or to the food once served, and 60–79 per cent during food processing or manufacture. Foods high in sodium chloride include ham, bacon, smoked fish, foods canned in brine, cheese, butter, salted nuts and biscuits and yeast extract. Significant contributions are also made because of the amount of bread, breakfast cereal, ready meats, canned meats, savoury snacks, soups and sauces consumed on a regular basis.

Main functions: The regulation of body water content, the maintenance of acid–base balance, blood volume and blood pressure, and nerve and muscle function.

Deficiency: Unlikely in normal circumstances.

Requirements: The RNI for adult men and women is 1,600mg per day for sodium, and 2,500mg per day for chloride. The Food Standards Agency and UK Health Departments advise to keep intakes at or below 6g salt a day.

Excessive intakes: The evidence for a direct association between salt intake and high blood pressure is now much stronger than was previously thought.

Potassium

Major food sources: Present in all foods except fats, oils and sugar. Particularly good sources are fruits (bananas and oranges), vegetables, potatoes, coffee, tea and cocoa.

Main functions: The regulation of fluid balance in conjunction with sodium. Potassium maintains water inside the cells (intracellular fluid), and sodium maintains water outside the cells (extracellular fluid). It appears to have a positive effect in reducing blood pressure (a reason to maintain fruit and vegetable intakes), and is involved in nerve and muscle function.

Deficiency: Unlikely. It can result from severe diarrhoea and vomiting.

Requirements: The RNI for adult men and women is 3,500mg per day.

Excessive intakes: Toxicity is only likely to occur by supplementation.

Iron

Major food sources: Liver, lean meat (especially red meat), kidney, heart, shellfish and egg yolks. Wholegrain cereals, dried pulses and dried fruit contain iron, but it is less well absorbed than iron from animal foods. Some breakfast cereals are fortified with iron. Vitamin C helps the absorption of iron from plant foods.

Main function: Iron is a part of the haemoglobin in red blood cells that carries oxygen to all parts of the body.

Deficiency: Low haemoglobin levels cause tiredness and fatigue, and ultimately iron deficiency anaemia. Iron deficiency is one of the most common nutritional deficiencies in developed and developing countries; as many as one in three women of child-bearing age in the UK is iron deficient.

Requirement: The RNI for women (eleven to fifty-plus years) is 14.8mg per day, and that for adult men is 8.7mg per day. The RNI for women is higher to make up for iron losses due to monthly periods.

Excessive intakes: There is no risk from normal foods other than in people with rare metabolic disorders.

Zinc
Major food sources: Red meat, liver, shellfish (especially oysters), dairy products and eggs. Wholegrain cereals, bread and pulses contain zinc, but it is less well absorbed.

Main functions: Zinc is a part of many enzymes needed for a variety of body functions involved in energy production, aiding wound healing, in the development of the body's immune system (antioxidant function) and in insulin production.

Deficiency: Insufficient zinc can slow down growth and development. It also delays wound healing, and may impair the immune function.

Requirement: The RNI for adult men is 9.5mg per day, and for adult women 7.0mg per day.

Excessive intakes: The acute ingestion of 2g of zinc produces nausea and vomiting. Long-term intakes of 50mg per day interfere with copper metabolism.

Copper
Major food sources: Present in trace quantities in many foods.

Main functions: Part of many enzyme systems, particularly those involved in metabolism and antioxidant function.

Deficiency: May have a role in the development of heart disease, but more research is needed.

Requirement: RNI for adult men and women is 1.2mg per day.

Excessive intakes: High intakes are toxic, but these only occur in abnormal circumstances such as contaminated water.

Selenium
Major food sources: Wholegrain cereals, meat, fish and shellfish, milk and egg yolks and Brazil nuts. The selenium content of food is dependent on the amount in the soil.

Main function: Powerful antioxidant (protects cell membranes).

Deficiency: There is no clinical condition associated with a dietary deficiency, but a possible link with the development of heart disease.

Requirements: The RNI for adult men is 75µg per day, and for adult women 60µg per day.

Excessive intakes: High levels (in excess of 1mg) are known to be toxic, and an upper limit of 6µg per kg per day for adults has been set.

Fluoride
Major food sources: Drinking water with a high natural or added fluoride level, fluoride toothpaste, fish and tea.

Main function: Bone and tooth mineralization, and helping in the prevention of tooth decay.

Deficiency: Increased susceptibility to tooth decay and lack of bone strength.

Requirements: No RNI set.

Excessive intakes: Causes mottling of the teeth.

Iodine
Major food sources: The only natural rich source is seafood. Other sources are milk and milk products, and iodized salt.

Main function: The functioning of the thyroid, and formation of thyroid hormones.

Deficiency: The resulting deficiency of thyroid hormone leads to a low metabolic rate and lethargy.

Requirements: The RNI for adult men and women is 140µg per day.

Excessive intakes: Not usually a problem.

Manganese
Major food sources: Tea.

Main function: Component of many enzymes.

Deficiency: Unobserved except in experimental studies.

Requirements: No RNI set, but safe intakes are believed to lie above 1.4mg per day for adults.

Excessive intakes: One of the least toxic elements. Excess intakes are quickly excreted.

Chromium
Major food sources: Meat, wholegrain cereals, legumes, nuts and Brewers' yeast.

Main function: Formation of insulin and lipoprotein metabolism.

Deficiency: Unlikely on a normal mixed diet.

Requirements: No RNI set, but safe intakes are believed to lie above 25µg per day for adults.

Molybdenum
Major food sources: Trace amounts found in many foods.

Main function: Enzyme function.

Deficiency: Reported on very low intakes (25µg per day) where the typical UK diet provides a mean of 128µg per day

Requirements: No RNI set, but safe intakes are believed to lie between 50 and 400µg per day.

Antioxidant Nutrients

Antioxidant nutrients are a group of vitamins, minerals and plant substances variously called phytochemicals, bioactive compounds or phytoprotectants, which act as defences against certain diseases. When oxygen is used in chemical reactions in the body it produces potentially harmful chemicals as by-products called free radicals. These free radicals are unstable molecules because they have part of their structure missing. They try to replace the missing bit by 'stealing' from other molecules, which can cause damage to tissues in the body and, amongst other things, may eventually cause heart disease and some cancers. The body has powerful defence mechanisms to prevent this damage occurring, but this can be impaired by environmental pollutants such as cigarette smoke, car fumes and excessive exposure to sunlight. Antioxidants can neutralize free radicals by giving up the missing part to the free radical without becoming unstable themselves.

The antioxidant vitamins are A, C and E; minerals with antioxidant properties include zinc, iron, copper and selenium. Phytochemicals found particularly in fruit and vegetables also act as antioxidants and include lycopene (tomatoes), saponins (onions), allicin (garlic) and indoles (broccoli, cabbage and Brussels sprouts). The advice to eat at least five portions of fruit and vegetables every day is partly because of the strong evidence that these foods are such powerful antioxidants.

THE WHOLE DIET APPROACH

Enjoying a diet that contains a wide variety of different foods can ensure that daily requirements for all the essential nutrients are met. A diet built around a very limited choice of foods, or one that is consistently low in overall food intake, will not. The simplest way to ensure that the basic diet contains all the essential nutrients is to follow the guidance of the Food Standards Agency's eatwell plate.

The eatwell plate

Putting foods into groups according to the main nutrients they supply makes it easier to choose wisely but enjoyably. Those who eat

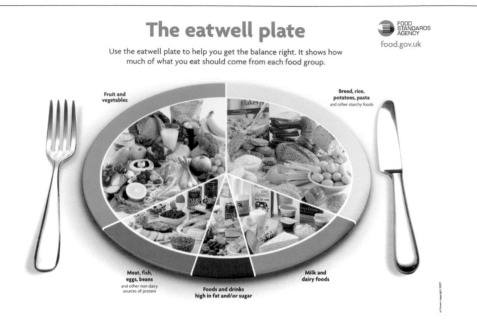

The eatwell plate, Food Standards Agency. © Crown copyright material is reproduced with the permission of the Controller of HMSO and Queen's Printer for Scotland.

the correct proportions of foods from the main food groups every day, and vary the choices within each group, will be eating well and therefore probably performing better. The actual amount eaten will of course depend on individual energy and nutrient requirements, but *The Balance of Good Health* provides an excellent foundation on which to build the training diet.

FROM PLATE TO MUSCLES

A quick tour through digestion and absorption shows how food is changed into a form that the body can use to keep itself healthy, to provide energy to fuel training and matches, and materials for muscle growth.

Chewing in the mouth begins to break down food mechanically. Saliva mixes with the food, making it easier to swallow, and an enzyme in it makes a start on digesting any carbohydrate. Saliva helps to protect against tooth decay. Once swallowed, the food passes down the oesophagus, reaching the stomach in about three seconds. A small amount of digestion takes place here, but the main function of the stomach is to break down the food mechanically and to kill any bacteria present in the food.

Food remains in the stomach between one and four hours, and small amounts are released into the small intestine. Foods rich in carbohydrate pass through faster than high fat foods, and liquids usually pass more quickly than food. Stress and nerves before a match can reduce the rate of gastric emptying.

The small intestine is made up of the duodenum, jejunum and ileum, and this is where most of the digestion and absorption processes take place. Bile produced in the liver and stored in the gall bladder breaks down fat into tiny droplets, making digestion more efficient. Pancreatic juices neutralize the acidic stomach contents, break down fats into fatty acids, proteins into peptides and amino acids, and starch into maltose. Finally, intestinal juices produced in the walls of the small intestine finish the breakdown of carbohydrates into the simple sugars glucose, fructose and galactose. What is left then passes into the large intestine (the colon, rectum and anus), where water used during digestion is reabsorbed.

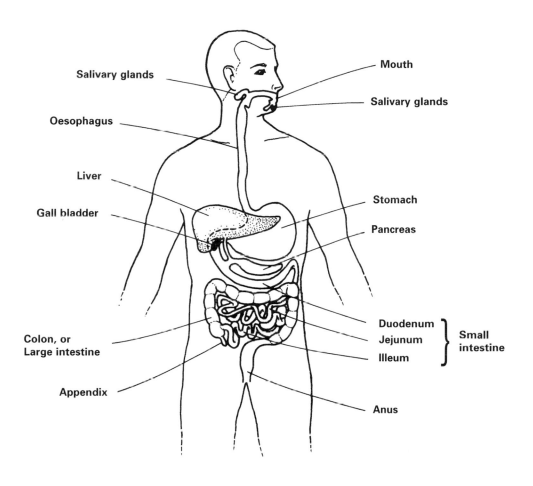

The digestive system.

Only a small amount of food passes through the system completely undigested, as bacteria in the colon finally get to work on fibre residues such as cellulose, breaking them down by fermentation to gases and fatty acids. More water is reabsorbed, and the residue (now called faeces) becomes drier and more solid as it passes along the rectum to the anus. It normally takes one to three days for food to complete the whole process from mouth to anus. (This can be checked personally by eating sweetcorn!) Most of the absorption of nutrients takes place through the walls of the small intestine, though small amounts of water, alcohol and soluble vitamins (B and C) and minerals (salt) can pass through the stomach lining into the bloodstream. The end products of digestion that are finally absorbed are peptides and amino acids from proteins, fatty acids from fats and glucose, fructose and galactose from carbohydrates.

ENERGY PRODUCTION

Both codes of rugby provide perfect examples of 'stop and go' sports. During matches players can be standing still, walking or jogging one minute, and sprinting, tackling, scrummaging or jumping the next. This switch from low intensity exercise to high intensity exercise puts demands on the skeletal muscles to respond quickly to changes in

The Five Food Groups

Bread, other Cereals and Potatoes

Bread, potatoes, pasta and noodles, rice, breakfast cereals. Other cereal grains such as oats, maize, millet and cornmeal, and starchy vegetables such as yams and plantains. Beans, peas and lentils can be included in this group, too.

They provide carbohydrate, dietary fibre, some calcium and iron, and B vitamins, and they are predominantly low in fat.

It is recommended to make these the main part of the diet.

Fruit and Vegetables

These include fresh, frozen and canned fruit and vegetables, and salad vegetables. Dried fruit and fruit juice can make up some of the choices.

These provide vitamins, particularly C, beta-carotene and folic acid, other antioxidants, dietary fibre and some carbohydrate. The darker the vegetables (broccoli, spinach, greens and peppers), the more beta-carotene is present. Fruit juice counts as only one portion, however much is drunk in a day. Beans and pulses can be eaten as part of this group, but only count as one portion, however much is eaten in a day.

It is recommended to eat at least five portions a day.

Milk and Dairy Foods

Milk, cheese, yogurt and fromage frais. This group does not include butter, eggs and cream.

These provide protein, calcium, vitamin B12, and the vitamins A and D (lower fat versions contain less of these fat-soluble vitamins).

Eat or drink in moderate amounts, and choose lower fat versions whenever possible.

Meat, Fish and Alternatives

Meat, poultry, fish, eggs, nuts, beans, peas and lentils. Includes bacon, salami and meat products such as sausages, beefburgers and pâté. Includes frozen and canned fish such as fish fingers, fish cakes, tuna and sardines.

These provide protein, iron and the B vitamins, especially B12, zinc and magnesium. Beans, peas and lentils also provide dietary fibre.

Eat moderate amounts and choose lower fat versions whenever possible.

Foods containing Fat; Foods and Drinks containing Sugar

Fat: Margarine, butter and other spreading fats (including low fat spreads), cooking oils, oil-based salad dressings, mayonnaise, cream, chocolate, crisps, biscuits, pastries, cakes, puddings, ice cream, rich sauces and gravies.

These provide fat, essential fatty acids, and some vitamins.

Eat foods containing fat sparingly, and look out for the low fat alternatives.

Sugar: Soft drinks, sweets, jam, honey, marmalade, biscuits, pastries, cakes, puddings, ice cream.

These provide carbohydrate, some minerals and vitamins, and fat in some products (but not others).

Foods and drinks containing sugar should not be consumed too often.

---

energy needs. All muscle activity is fuelled by the chemical adenosine triphosphate (ATP), which is produced in the body by three energy systems: the aerobic system breaks down or oxidizes carbohydrate and fat to produce ATP; the phosphagen system produces short-term energy in the form of ATP and creatine phosphate; and the anaerobic glycolytic system breaks down glycogen (stored carbohydrate) in the muscles to ATP and lactic acid.

The phosphagen system provides energy for explosive movements or short bursts of activity. Only small quantities of creatine phosphate are stored in the muscles, enough to sustain high intensity movement for about 10sec. The anaerobic system provides energy for limited periods of 2 to 3min of high intensity work. Accumulation of the by-product lactic acid leads to muscle fatigue, which limits performance drastically. Periods of low

The Fate of Major Nutrients in the Body

Carbohydrates
- Transported to all cells; energy provision.
- Converted into glycogen; stored in the liver and muscles; readily available energy source.
- Converted into fatty acids; stored as body fat; potential energy source.

Fats: Rebuilt into triglycerides; carried by lymphatic system to blood; stored as body fat; triglycerides stored in muscle.

Proteins: Amino acids carried to the liver; join the amino acid pool in the circulation; converted into other amino acids; oxidized for energy often after conversion into glucose, or converted and stored as fat.

The Energy Systems

$$ATP \rightarrow ADP + P \text{ (phosphate)} + Energy$$

Aerobic energy system
$$Glucose/fatty\ acids + oxygen \rightarrow ATP \rightarrow Energy + carbon\ dioxide + water$$

Phosphagen energy system
$$ADP + CP \text{ (creatine phosphate)} \rightarrow C \text{ (creatine)} + ATP \rightarrow Energy$$

Anaerobic glycolytic system
$$ADP + glucose \rightarrow ATP + lactic\ acid \rightarrow Energy$$

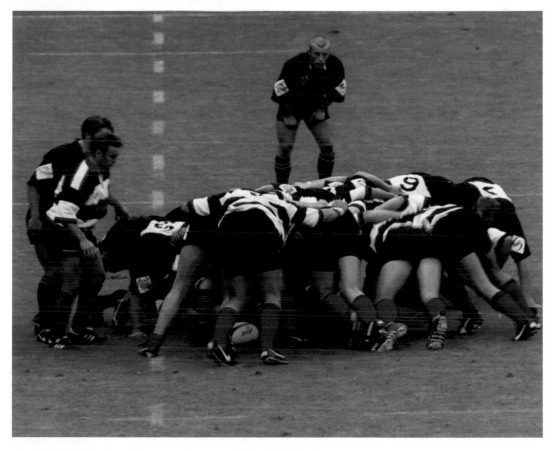

Scrum, aerial view; Wasps v. Saracens. (© PA Photos)

Running Intensities

Varying running intensities by position and tackle and ruck counts during a 2003 international rugby match (courtesy of RFU 2003)

	Prop	flanker	fly half	centre	wing
Sprinting (min-sec)	0:0	0:03	0:27	0:19	0.31
High-speed running (min-sec)	0:27	1:08	2:36	1:25	1:44
Running (min-sec)	5:35	5:56	5:10	3:36	3:42
Jogging (min-sec)	16:06	13:36	14:34	14:45	12:42
Walking (min-sec)	56:38	51:10	47:21	54:45	57:01
Tackles	15	25	15	12	9
Rucks	40	46	22	22	16

intensity exercise such as walking, jogging or just resting provide opportunities to convert lactic acid into less toxic substances for removal via the bloodstream.

The aerobic pathway produces ATP, with oxygen and carbohydrate and fat as the main dietary fuels. This system has the advantage of producing energy for 2 to 3min up to several hours, and therefore fuels all medium to low intensity exercise. Carbon dioxide and water produced as by-products are absorbed into the bloodstream and removed. Although emphasis is placed on the importance of maintaining fuel supplies for the constantly changing physical demands, the cognitive aspects must not be forgotten. Diet plays an important part in mental as well as physical performance in both training and matches.

CHAPTER 2

The Training Diet

The training diet is basically what players eat on a day-to-day basis to support their training programme, to help their recovery from all training sessions, to minimize fatigue and keep their bodies healthy. In order to build up their diet, players will need to have some idea of their total daily energy, carbohydrate and protein requirements. They will also need to know the best way to fuel up before a training session, how to refuel effectively after training sessions, and how to manipulate the energy and nutrient balance to increase muscle mass or lose body fat or both. To keep the body healthy a player will need to know which foods to include and in what amounts to ensure an optimal intake of key minerals and vitamins. Of course, having the knowledge is only half the mission: the other half is to know how to put this theory into practice every day.

ENERGY REQUIREMENTS

The basal metabolic rate (BMR) and the energy cost of all activities account for almost the total daily energy requirement. The BMR is the amount of energy needed when the body is fasting and at complete rest – in other words, the energy needed for all the bodily functions including respiration, digestion and metabolism. Several factors affect the BMR: it decreases with age, is lower in women (because of their higher proportion of body fat), and higher when there is a greater proportion of muscle. The BMR accounts for 60 to 75 per cent of total energy expenditure in people with sedentary lifestyles where activity level is very low.

Having established the BMR, the cost of the daily activities must now be calculated. The simplest method is based on the physical

Calculating the Basal Metabolic Rate		
(*See* References, Chapter 2, 1.)		
Age	BMR (males)	BMR (females)
10–17yr	$17.7 \times W + 657$	$13.4 \times W + 692$
18–29yr	$15.1 \times W + 692$	$14.8 \times W + 487$
30–59yr	$11.5 \times W + 873$	$8.3 \times W + 846$
W = bodyweight (kg)		

For example:
For a 22-year-old player weighing 100kg:
$BMR = 15.1 \times 100 + 692 \rightarrow 2202kcals$

activity level (PAL). Players must make an assumption of the energy demands of their job or occupation, and of the rest of the day (non-occupational activity), to establish their PAL. Having determined the most appropriate PAL, the estimated energy requirement (EAR) can then be calculated.

CARBOHYDRATE REQUIREMENTS

The training diet must provide sufficient carbohydrate for a player to refuel effectively after every training session and match. Carbohydrate is the primary fuel for muscle contraction for endurance, strength and speed. Unfortunately the body can only store a limited amount of carbohydrate as glycogen in the muscles and liver. As exercise intensity increases, the energy demand met by carbohydrate breakdown increases. During weights and sprinting sessions players will rely almost exclusively on carbohydrate for their fuel source, yet muscle glycogen stores can be depleted after only 15 to 30 minutes at very high exercise intensities (90 to 130 per cent VO_{2max}). Intense training loads therefore place heavy demands on carbohydrate reserves, which must be replaced.

Calculated Physical Activity Levels

The table below shows the calculated physical activity level (PAL) of adults at three levels each of occupational and non-occupational activity.

Non-Occupational Activity	Occupational Activity					
	Light		Moderate		Moderate/Heavy	
	M	F	M	F	M	F
Non-active	1.4	1.4	1.6	1.5	1.7	1.5
Moderately active	1.5	1.5	1.7	1.6	1.8	1.6
Very active	1.6	1.6	1.8	1.7	1.9	1.7

For example: A 22-year-old rugby player weighing 100kg has a light job but a very active lifestyle:

$$BMR = 15.1 \times 100 + 692 = 2,202$$
$$PAL = 1.6$$
$$EAR = BMR \times PAL = 2,202 \times 1.6 = 3,523 kcal/d$$

Carbohydrate Requirements

Moderate daily recovery and match preparation	5–7g per kg bodyweight per day
Enhanced daily recovery and match preparation i.e. heavy training (twice a day)	7–12g per kg bodyweight per day
For immediate recovery after training/matches	1.0–1.2g per kg

Note: Requirements will vary over the week, season and even playing years, and intake will need to be adjusted to match them.

individual. Some players may still prefer to refuel immediately and so be able to 'tick the box'. This may apply particularly to young players. The advantages of including protein with carbohydrate post-exercise are discussed in the chapter on muscle gain.

Chronic glycogen depletion will reduce a player's ability to recover from, and respond to, a heavy training programme. The more training sessions undertaken in a week, and particularly in a day, the more a player will have to recover within hours rather than days. Restocking glycogen stores is essential, but this can only be achieved by players including enough carbohydrate in their diet on a daily basis, and paying particular attention to their refuelling immediately after all training sessions and matches.

The restocking of muscle glycogen stores is greatest during the first hour after exercise. If there are fewer than eight hours between training sessions, players should consume carbohydrate as soon as they can after the first session to maximize recovery before the start of the next one. This can be achieved by an immediate post-training refueller, including a sports drink followed by a meal. However, some players may prefer to eat and drink 'little and often' (every 15 to 30min) rather than have a meal. When recovery time is twenty-four hours or longer, recovery can be achieved by an eating pattern that suits the

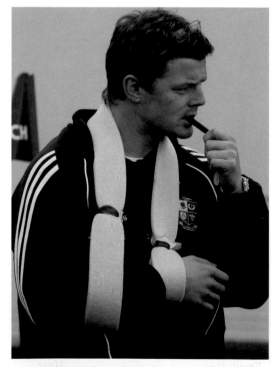

Injured British and Lions captain Brian O'Driscoll eats confectionary as his team-mates train in New Zealand. (© PA Photos)

Good Sources of Carbohydrate

- Cereals: Any variety including hot cereals such as porridge. Many varieties can be eaten dry as a quick snack.
- Bread: All types including bagels, English muffins, crumpets, pikelets, naans, chappatis, potato cakes, raisin bread, malt loaf, fruit loaf, rye bread, tea breads, pancakes, Scotch pancakes, tortillas and wraps, soft pretzels.
- Fruit muffins and fruit bread.
- Crispbreads, water biscuits, oatcakes, crackers, rice cakes and matzos.
- Pasta and noodles.
- Rice.
- Polenta, couscous, oatmeal, bulgur wheat, millet and quinoa.
- Potatoes, sweet potatoes, yam, cassava, plantains.
- Pizza bases (thick base if possible).
- Beans: Baked, butter, red kidney, barlotti, cannelloni and mixed.
- Peas, lentils, pearl barley, chickpeas.
- Sweetcorn.
- Root vegetables: Carrots, parsnips, swedes, turnips, sweet potatoes, beetroot.
- Fruit: Fresh, dried, canned, cooked.
- Jam, marmalade, honey, fruit spreads, golden syrup, maple syrup, molasses, black treacle.
- Twiglets, sesame sticks, Japanese rice crackers, breadsticks, pretzels.
- Biscuits: Jaffa cakes, fig rolls, garibaldi, rich tea, plain digestives.
- Cakes: Currant buns, tea cakes, iced buns, Chelsea buns, plain or fruit scones, fruit cake and fruit loaf, gingerbread, parkin, jam-filled Swiss roll, flapjacks and other similar 'simple or plain' cakes.
- Breakfast, cereal, muesli and cake bars.
- Puddings: Fruit crumbles, bread pudding, milk puddings (e.g. rice pudding and Müller Rice), pancakes, jelly and custard, banana and custard, meringues, ice cream.
- Yogurt: Fruit and natural.
- Milk, flavoured milk, milk shakes and smoothies.
- Sweetened soft drinks: Squash, cordial, canned drinks.
- Fruit juice and vegetable juice.
- Popcorn (preferably salted, not buttered).
- Confectionery: Chocolate bars and sweets e.g. jelly babies, wine gums and M&S Percy Pigs.
- Sugar: Added to drinks and breakfast cereals.
- Sports products: Drinks, bars and gels.

Portions of food providing approx 50g carbohydrate*

	Weight (approx)	Household measure
Breakfast cereals		
Porridge oats	75g (uncooked weight)	5 tablespoons
Wholewheat biscuits	65g	3–4 biscuits
Muesli	70g	5 tablespoons
Cornflake-type cereals	60g	10 tablespoons
Breads and bakery goods		
Bread, large, medium sliced	100g	3 slices
Bread, large, thick sliced	100g	2½ slices
Bagel	70g	1

continued overleaf

Good Sources of Carbohydrate *continued*

Rolls	100g	2
Baps (very large rolls)	100g	1
Pitta bread, large	95g	1
Crumpets	125g	3
Fruit scone	100g	2
Currant buns	100g	2
Malt loaf	100g	2½ slices
Cereals and grains		
Pasta (cooked)	225g (70g uncooked)	8 tablespoons
Rice (cooked)	175g (60g uncooked)	4 heaped tablespoons
Pizza base (thick)	½ large (9in)	
Potatoes		
Boiled	300g	5 egg-sized
Jacket	175g	1 medium (with skin)
Mashed	325g	7 heaped tablespoons
Oven chips	175g	approximately 20
Dairy		
Semi-skimmed milk	1⅔ pints/950ml	
Fruit		
Apples		4 medium
Bananas		2 large
Dried apricots	100g	15
Dried dates	100g	7
Figs	100g	5
Raisins	70g	2½ tablespoons
Sultanas	70g	2½ tablespoons
Unsweetened orange juice	568ml/1 pint	

* Information about manufactured products can be found on the food labels.

Practical Ways to Boost Carbohydrate Intake

- Eat frequently! Have regular meals, mini meals and refuellers throughout the day.
- Base every eating occasion around a carbohydrate-rich food. Make it the biggest portion of the meal.
- Use thick-sliced bread rather than medium- or thin-sliced.
- Have bread as well as pasta, rice or potatoes with meals on hard training days.
- Jam, marmalade, honey and fruit spreads provide carbohydrate but no fat. They should be spread thickly and the fat thinly.
- Boiled, mashed or jacket potatoes are low in fat, chips are not. Thick-cut oven varieties are the best chip choice.
- Sweet potatoes, plantains and cassava can make an interesting change to potatoes.
- Rice is not difficult to cook, but brown rice is easier and parboiled easiest, though more expensive. Cook rice in bulk and freeze portions. Frozen rice can be reheated in a minute in a microwave.
- Use different shapes of pasta to relieve boredom. Melted low fat soft cheese

makes a very quick pasta sauce to which cooked chicken, ham or canned tuna can be added.

- Extra pasta or rice can be turned into a lunch the following day.
- Get out of the pasta rut and experiment with bulgur wheat, couscous and polenta – all available in pre-cooked forms.
- Breakfast cereals can be eaten at any time, even just before bed.
- Breakfast cereal and fruit juice complement each other. Both provide carbohydrate, and the vitamin C in the juice helps iron absorption from the cereal.
- Red kidney beans, borlotti beans, cannelloni beans, chickpeas and sweetcorn can be added to canned vegetable or minestrone soups, to tomato sauces with pasta, and to curry sauces with rice. They all add protein to the meal, too.
- Baked beans on toast makes a quick and easy meal, again providing carbohydrate and protein. Warm pitta bread can be used for a change.
- Frozen pitta bread can be warmed from frozen quickly in a toaster or under the grill.
- Add fresh (especially bananas), canned or dried fruit to breakfast cereal; have canned fruit and low fat custard; or try a banana sandwich.
- Low fat milkshakes (e.g. semi-skimmed milk, low fat yogurt and a banana) or just an extra pint of semi-skimmed milk will provide quality protein, too.

THE GI FACTOR

The glycaemic index (GI factor) is a ranking of foods based on the rate at which a food raises blood glucose level. All foods are compared to a reference food, either glucose or white bread using the amount of food needed to provide 50g carbohydrate. This gives a measure of how quickly a carbohydrate-rich food is digested and absorbed. This can obviously have practical implications when considering what to have before training/matches and for immediate refuelling afterwards. However, the GI does not give the complete picture, as it does not take into account the amount of carbohydrate in a portion. Parsnips have a high GI, but this will have been based on a weight of 400g (the amount providing 50g carbohydrate): an average portion of parsnips is 65g and only contains 8g, which would have little or no glycaemic effect. The glycaemic load (GL) takes portion sizes into consideration.

Carbohydrate-rich foods with a moderate to high GI appear to be better choices for restocking muscle glycogen stores than low GI foods. Contrary to popular belief, research has shown that it is not necessary to keep to low GI food before exercise. Sports drinks have a high GI, which makes them appropriate for before, during and immediately after exercise.

The Glycaemic Index of Some Common Foods

Low GI foods (GI less than 55)
Noodles, pasta, basmati rice, lentils; apples and apple juice, pears, oranges and orange juice, grapes, bananas, dried apricots; milk, low fat yogurt; fruit loaf; baked beans; porridge, 'fruit and fibre'-type cereals; granary and multigrain breads.

Intermediate GI foods (GI 55–70)
New and boiled potatoes, macaroni, couscous; pineapple, sultanas and raisins; pitta bread, fibre-enriched white bread, oatmeal biscuits; and honey.

High GI factor foods (GI more than 70)
Instant and mashed potato, jacket potatoes and chips, brown and white rice, parsnips, swede, broad beans and watermelon; cornflakes, Weetabix, Shredded Wheat and Rice Krispies; brown, wholemeal, and brown and white bread; bagels, crumpets and rice cakes; jelly babies and jelly beans.

There are many books covering the topic of GI, which give a wider selection of foods and their GI values. An international table of GI and GL values has also been published. (*See* References Chapter 2, 2)

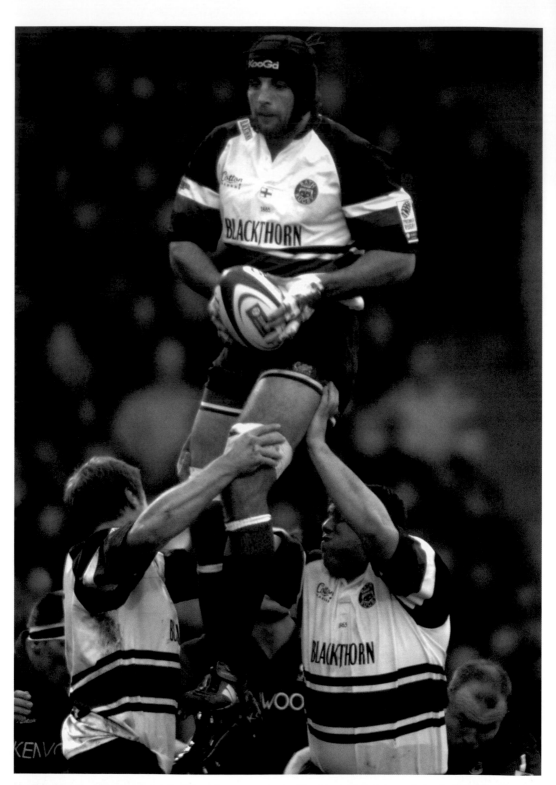

Bath's Danny Grewcock (c) is lifted by team-mates Duncan Bell (r) and Andy Beattie (l) to claim the ball in the lineout. (© PA Photos)

PROTEIN IN THE DIET

Protein requirements are 1.4–1.7g per kg bodyweight per day, taking into account both the strength and endurance elements of the game. If the training programme is weighted more towards strength training, players should aim for the upper end of the range. People with a sedentary lifestyle or very low levels of activity have a requirement of 0.75g protein per kg bodyweight per day.

This could lead some players to believe that they need to make enormous efforts to increase their intake, including the use of protein supplements. However, the general population more than meets its requirements, and with the increased consumption of food to meet energy needs, players will probably meet their requirements without having to resort to supplements. Players who include protein and carbohydrate at all their meals, who maintain their bodyweight and have enough energy to meet their training demands, can be confident that their diet is providing the right amount of protein.

The timing of protein intakes around training sessions is important, especially those sessions designed to aid muscle gain. This is covered in some detail in Chapter 5, where portions of foods providing 20g protein are included. Even in these situations it is perfectly feasible for most players to meet their requirements without the use of protein and amino acid supplements.

Can a Player Have Too Much Protein?

Intakes under 2g per kg bodyweight in healthy players are unlikely to cause any side effects. High intakes may increase the overall energy intake above requirements, which could lead to an increase in body fat, or they could push out other foods from the diet resulting in a reduction in intake of essential nutrients obtained from non-protein foods. Intakes above 3g per kg bodyweight may have a number of negative effects including kidney damage, increased blood lipoprotein levels (associated with atherosclerosis) and dehydration.

FAT IN THE DIET

Although players have high energy requirements, this cannot be used as an excuse to indulge in high intakes of fat. Fat stored as adipose tissue is a source of fuel, but only for the lightest intensity exercise or very prolonged endurance exercise. The priority fuel is carbohydrate. Fat intake can be kept to sensible amounts by observing the following suggestions.

Practical Hints for Controlling Fat Intake

- Choose a low fat spread rather than butter, hard margarine or soft margarine, but still spread it thinly (particularly as several slices of bread may be eaten a day).
- It may not be necessary to use anything on bread or toast – for example, baked beans on toast, peanut butter or honey sandwiches.
- Semi-skimmed milk not only has less fat, but more protein and calcium than whole milk.
- Either use reduced fat cheeses, or less of a strongly flavoured cheese.
- Grate cheese for sandwiches or toasted cheese – it goes further.
- Use low fat or reduced fat salad cream or mayonnaise when possible.
- Make 'creamy' sauces by gently melting low fat soft cheese.
- Cut down on crisps, chocolate, pastries and 'rich' cakes and biscuits. Snack on carbohydrate foods such as fruit (fresh or dried), sandwiches with low fat fillings, 'plain' cakes and biscuits (currant buns, scones, tea bread, crumpets, Rich Tea biscuits, fig rolls, plain digestives, Jaffa cakes).
- Eat fish more often – but grilled, microwaved, steamed or baked rather than deep-fried in batter.
- Grill fish cakes and fish fingers, too.
- Chicken and turkey are low in fat, especially if the skin is not eaten. Most of the fat is found underneath and comes off when the skin is removed (before or after cooking).

- Buy the leanest, affordable cuts of meat and trim off any visible fat (before or after cooking).
- Use any cooking method other than frying.
- Meat products such as sausages or beefburgers can be fatty, so do not eat them too often.
- Meat pies, sausage rolls and pasties contain a lot of fat in the meat and the pastry, so limit intake of these foods as much as possible.
- Keep pastry to one layer – the top or bottom crust only.
- Measure out oil when cooking rather than just pouring from the container.
- Stir-frying needs hardly any oil.
- Use non-stick pans to cut down the need for oil (and make washing-up easier, too).
- Flavour foods with low oil dressings, lemon or lime juice, balsamic vinegar, tomato ketchup or mustard.
- Thick oven chips are the best chip choice (5 per cent sunflower oil).
- Keep junk/fast food to a minimum.

High fat diets are associated with an increased risk of heart disease, stroke, some forms of cancer, and of course of becoming overweight and even obese. High fat diets also suppress some aspects of immune function compared to carbohydrate-rich diets. There is, however, one group of high fat foods that should be included in the weekly diet: oily fish. These contain the omega-3 fatty acids that are thought not only to have an impact on heart health, but also to have an important role in brain and eye function as well as a potential to relieve symptoms of stiffness and pain in joints. The recommendation is to have two portions (280g) of oily fish a week, which means including in the diet salmon (but not canned), canned sardines, herring, mackerel, fresh tuna and trout.

MINERALS, SALT AND ANTIOXIDANTS

The three minerals calcium, iron and selenium need to be considered specifically because

Reference Nutrient Intakes for Calcium, Iron and Selenium			
Males	*Calcium*	*Iron*	*Selenium*
11–14 years	1,000mg	11.3mg	45µg
15–18 years	1,000mg	11.3mg	70µg
19–50 years	700mg	8.7mg	75µg
Females			
11–14 years	800mg	14.5mg	45µg
15–18 years	800mg	14.8mg	60µg
19–50 years	700mg	14.8mg	60µg

they could be lacking in the diet and so affect performance or health.

Calcium

Almost 90 per cent of calcium is found in the bones. Bone is an active tissue, constantly changing as a result of the continual process of bone resorption and bone formation. Peak bone mass is the highest bone mass that is achieved in a person's lifetime, and is normally reached by the early thirties. After this time, bone mass begins to fall with age as resorption starts to exceed formation slightly. The rate of decline in bone mass with age is similar regardless of the peak bone mass achieved, so having a high peak bone mass will help to prevent or at least delay the onset of osteoporosis in later life. Dairy products are the best source of calcium, yet many people have cut down or even cut out milk from their diets.

Practical Ways to Increase Calcium Intake
One of the easiest ways to ensure an adequate intake is to consume 'Three-A-Day': an average glass (200ml) of semi-skimmed or skimmed milk, a small pot (150g) of low fat yogurt, and a matchbox-sized (40g) piece of cheese. Having milk or yogurt with breakfast cereal every morning can boost the absorption of calcium from cereal, too.

Other simple ways to boost intake include adding grated cheese to salads, soups and home-made pizzas; sprinkling sesame or sunflower seeds on salads and cooked vegetables, using yogurt-based dressings on salads, and

Good Sources of Calcium in the Diet	
Dairy produce:	
1 pint whole milk	673mg*
1 pint semi-skimmed milk	702mg
1 pint skimmed milk	702mg
Matchbox-size piece of Cheddar (40g)	288mg
Matchbox-size piece low fat Cheddar (40g)	336mg
4oz/100g cottage cheese	73mg
5oz/150g pot fruit yogurt	225mg
1 pint soya non-dairy alternative with calcium	505mg
Cereals:	
2 large slices white or brown bread	80mg
2 large slices wholemeal bread	39mg
Fish:	
100g can sardines in tomato sauce (with bones)	460mg
¼ 418g can salmon	313mg
60g shelled prawns (average 20)	90mg
Vegetables and pulses:	
3 'spears' of broccoli (150g)	50mg
Quarter of a bunch watercress	34mg
2 tablespoons (90g) cooked spinach	144mg
225g can baked beans in tomato sauce	120mg
2 tablespoons canned red kidney beans (70g)	50mg
Average serving tofu (bean curd)	306mg
Nuts and seeds:	
100g bag plain peanuts	60mg
50g almonds	120mg
50g hazelnuts	70mg
1 tablespoon sesame seeds	80mg
Fruit:	
12 ready-to-eat dried apricots	73mg
5 dried figs	250mg
1 large orange	50mg
Ice cream and chocolate:	
1 scoop dairy ice cream	78mg
Standard bar milk chocolate (54g)	119mg
Standard bar white chocolate (66g)	178mg

* Calcium is present in the *non*-fat part of milk, therefore a pint of semi-skimmed milk contains more than a pint of whole milk.

topping jacket potatoes with natural yogurt and chives. Porridge can be made with milk rather than water. Custard made with milk can be enjoyed with fruit, alone or as a frozen dessert. Mashing up canned salmon or sardines, including the calcium-rich bones, with lemon juice provides a variation on tuna for a sandwich filling. Baked beans can be used as a vegetable, not just for beans on toast. Refuelling after training with milk shakes and smoothies made with milk, yogurt and fruit will boost calcium intake, and a mug of hot chocolate made with milk can give a final boost to the day's intake at bedtime.

Iron

Iron is found in haemoglobin in the red blood cells, in myoglobin in the muscle cells and in some of the oxidative enzymes in the mitochondria (the energy-producing factories in the cells). A shortage of iron will therefore have a serious effect on energy metabolism. A deficiency of iron is accompanied by common symptoms such as chronic fatigue, susceptibility to stress, increased susceptibility to infections and decreased cognitive performance. Sub-optimal iron status is one of the most common nutritional problems found in the general community.

Iron in the Diet

There are two types of iron in the diet: haem iron in meat and meat products, and non-haem iron in cereals, vegetables, peas, beans and lentils and fruits. Haem iron is well absorbed, up to 20 to 40 per cent being taken up, whereas only 5 to 20 per cent of iron from vegetable sources, egg and milk is absorbed. Many players avoid eating red meat, preferring to eat chicken instead. If the only reason is a preference, rather than a dislike of a meat, perhaps an appreciation of the amount of iron in red meat might encourage such players to include it in their diet once or twice a week.

Female players need to pay particular attention to their iron intake to ensure they replace the losses that occur through their monthly periods. In some cases regular daily intake of a vitamin and mineral supplement

Good Sources of Iron in the Diet

Animal sources:

2 slices liver (100g)	9mg
1 whole pig's kidney (140g)	9mg
1 portion black pudding (75g)	15mg
8oz/225g lean beef steak	6mg
4oz/100g lean minced beef	2.7mg
3 large beef sausages, grilled (120g)	1.7mg
2 thick slices corned beef	2.9mg
Pâté, low fat slice on bread (40g)	2.5mg
1 chicken breast	0.65mg
1 chicken quarter	2.0mg
1 small can tuna in brine	1.0mg
1 large fillet white fish	0.5mg
6 cockles	6.2mg
6 mussels	3.2mg
1 size 3 egg	1.1mg

Cereals:

2 slices white bread	1.0mg
2 slices wholemeal bread	1.9mg
Breakfast cereals*	
Pasta, cooked av. portion (7½ tbsp)	1.8mg
Rice, cooked av. portion (4½ tbsp)	0.4mg

Vegetables and pulses:

Average portion spinach	1.7mg
Large portion cabbage	0.7mg
Large portion peas	1.4mg
225g can baked beans in tomato sauce	3.2mg
120g cooked red lentils (3 tbsp)	2.9mg
120g cooked brown or green lentils (3 tbsp)	4.2mg
Average portion tofu (bean curd)	0.7mg

Nuts:

25g bag cashew nuts	1.6mg
1 tablespoon sesame seeds	1.1mg

Fruit:

12 ready-to-eat dried apricots	3.4mg
6 dried dates	1.0mg
2 tablespoons raisins	0.8mg
6 prunes	1.6mg

* Many breakfast cereals are enriched with iron. Check the nutritional information panel on the box.

that contains the RDI for iron might be beneficial.

Practical Ways to Increase Iron Intake

Breakfast cereals that are fortified with iron are a good choice, especially as they will probably be eaten once, if not sometimes twice a day in good amounts. Vitamin C helps the absorption of iron, particularly from non-haem iron foods, so including a glass of orange or grapefruit juice with breakfast cereals, adding tomatoes and peppers to sandwiches and cooked dishes, and drinking squashes containing added vitamin C with meals, can all help to boost intake. Strong tea and coffee should be drunk *between* meals, rather than with them, as the tannins present can reduce iron absorption. Bran and wheatgerm should also be avoided for similar reasons.

The absorption of iron from vegetables and cereals can be improved by eating a source of animal protein at the same meal. Wholegrain breads and cereals are better choices than those with added bran, as excessive bran intakes can reduce iron absorption. Non-meat eaters should ensure that their diet contains some of the following on a daily basis: wholegrain cereals and flours, nuts, dark green leafy vegetables, pulses, eggs, dried fruit and seeds (pumpkin, sesame, sunflower).

Selenium

Inclusion of foods high in selenium is important for brain function, and low levels in the body are associated with negative mood. Selenium intakes in the UK have been falling over the last thirty years, primarily because North American wheat, which has a high selenium content, is no longer imported, and has been replaced by low selenium EU and UK varieties.

Good Sources of Selenium in the Diet

Brazil nuts	3	25μg
Lamb's kidney, whole	1	73μg
Lamb's liver	100g	50μg
Crab, boiled	100g	84μg

Salt

Health professionals encourage a reduction in salt intake because of the possible link between regular high intakes and the development of high blood pressure. The average salt intake is 9.5g a day (equivalent to about two teaspoons), and the current recommendation is to reduce this to 6g a day. However, players do need to replace salt lost through sweating, in which case intakes should probably be kept slightly above this general public recommendation. The simplest way to increase salt intake when sweat losses have been high is to add it to meals at the table so that others who may be sharing the same meals can keep to a lower intake. The use of sports drinks is obviously another way to help replace losses.

Antioxidants

The simplest way to ensure that the body has plenty of antioxidants is to consume at least five portions of fruit and vegetables a day, making them as colourful and varied in colour as possible. In Australia five portions would not be considered enough, and native Australians aim for three to five portions of fruit and five to seven portions of vegetables. So what is a portion?

A 'Portion' Explained

Large fruit: Grapefruits, mangoes, melons, papayas and pineapples: one large slice.

Medium fruit: Apples, avocados, bananas, oranges, peaches, pears: one whole fruit.

Small fruit: Apricots, clementines, figs, kiwi fruit, passion fruit, plums, satsumas, tangerines and tomatoes: two whole fruit.

Very small fruit: Blackberries, blackcurrants, bilberries, cherries, cranberries, gooseberries, grapes, raspberries, strawberries: one cupful.

Fruit salad: Fresh, stewed or canned fruit: three tablespoons.

Dried fruit: Apricots, bananas, cranberries, currants, dates, figs, papaya, pineapple, raisins, sultanas: one tablespoon.

Fruit and vegetable juice: Freshly squeezed or processed juice, but not fruit drinks: one medium glass (150ml). Counts as one portion regardless of how many glasses are drunk.

Mixed salad vegetables: For example celery, cucumber, lettuce, peppers, tomatoes: one dessert bowlful.

Vegetables: Raw, cooked, frozen or canned: two tablespoons.

What doesn't count? Potatoes, yam, cassava, nuts and seeds, coconut, marmalade, jam, fruit 'drinks' and squashes do not count.

What does count? Fresh, frozen, canned, 100 per cent juice and dried fruit all count.

ALCOHOL

Drinking alcohol, sometimes to excess, is often seen as part of team bonding; certainly binge drinking occurs most often after matches. But what are the effects of alcohol on a player? After ingestion, some alcohol is quickly absorbed from the stomach, the remainder being absorbed lower down in the small intestine. After absorption, the blood alcohol level rises as the 'alcoholic blood' circulates around the body, acting first as a stimulant and then in some cases as a depressant. Eventually it is metabolized in the liver at the rate of about one unit an hour, after which the breakdown products can be used as a source of energy or converted into fat and stored.

Alcohol as a source of energy in exercise is limited – it is certainly not possible to 'work it off'. Quite apart from the serious long-term problems of regular, addictive heavy intakes that some high profile sportspeople have experienced, there are more common problems. First and foremost, an alcoholic drink is a concentrated source of calories *see* box below.

Average Energy Content of Alcoholic Drinks	
1 pint premium lager	300kcals
Pub measure vodka with a can Red Bull	150kcals
Alcopops (average per 275ml bottle)	180kcals
1 pint bitter	180kcals
Spirits (pub measure)	50kcals
Red wine (150ml)	85kcals
Dry white wine (150ml)	80kcals
Medium white wine (150ml	85kcals
Sweet white wine (150ml)	120kcals
Champagne (125ml)	95kcals

Second, the heavy drinker will feel 'hung over'. A hangover is usually caused by the dehydrating effects of alcohol, which acts as a diuretic, taking fluid from the body and increasing urine output (hence the need to get up in the small hours to go to the bathroom). The non-alcoholic congeners that give flavour, smell and colour to some drinks will also contribute to the symptoms of a hangover. The following are typical effects of increasing the blood alcohol level:

Two to three drinks in two hours (blood alcohol 20–40mg per litre):
Feel less tense and more relaxed.

Four to five drinks in two hours (blood alcohol now 60–90mg per litre):
Judgement, fine motor skills and co-ordination become impaired. Feelings of euphoria.

Six to nine drinks in two hours (110–160mg per litre):
Speech becomes slurred, motor co-ordination is seriously impaired and walking becomes staggered.

Nine to twelve drinks in two hours (180–250mg per litre):
Loss of control of voluntary activity, erratic behaviour and impaired vision (seeing double and objects moving around).

Thirteen to eighteen drinks in two hours (279–390mg per litre):
Probably unconscious with total loss of any co-ordination.

The Effects of Alcohol on Exercise

Alcohol has an adverse effect on reaction time, balance, concentration, hand/eye co-ordination, visual perception and the ability to make correct decisions. Any of these could increase the risk of serious injury from an accident or involvement in a fight. It may impair body temperature regulation during prolonged exercise in a cold environment.

Furthermore, heavy drinking could have a negative influence on performance the following day due to the effects of a hangover. Players do not perform at their best when dehydrated, depressed (a common symptom of a hangover, responsible for the 'I am never going to do this again' syndrome), and suffering headache and hypersensitivity to outside stimuli such as light and sound.

Alcohol can also slow injury recovery as it causes the blood vessels to the skin, arms and legs to open up. The increased blood supply makes an injury bleed and swell even more, and possibly slows the recovery process.

Managing Alcohol Intake

To eat before going out drinking is sound advice, as food in the stomach slows down the speed that alcohol gets into the bloodstream. Drinking slowly, and putting the glass down between mouthfuls rather than holding on to it and talking a lot, can help to keep the overall intake down – and so does avoiding having your drink topped up, in that you can then keep a check on how much you really are drinking. On getting home, rehydrating with plenty of water can go some way to preventing a hangover; it is a good idea to put a glass and jug of water by the bed before going out as a reminder.

MANAGING EATING AND TRAINING

Eating before Training

Food must be digested and absorbed before training begins. Foods high in fat and fibre take longest to be digested, as do larger meals generally. Low-intensity training sessions, or sessions such as swimming or cycling where the body is supported, are less likely to lead to discomfort in the stomach area than high-intensity sessions. As a general rule, a snack can be eaten one to two hours before a session, whereas three to four hours are needed between a meal and training. Players will need to work out what suits them best, but should remember that carbohydrate and fluids will probably be the key elements they will need to consider.

The GI of the pre-training meal or snack does not seem to matter. Though in theory a low GI meal would seem to be more beneficial because it would result in a slow and sustained release of glucose, research has not actually backed this up. Drinking a sports drink during training is an easy way of maintaining fuel levels.

Early morning training sessions can prove problematic for some players. Eating well the evening before is vital, as this will ensure the muscles are well stocked, and a snack an hour before training will top up the blood glucose level – a banana or cereal bar or a couple of pieces of toast may be enough for most players. Carbohydrate is needed not just for physical performance, but also for mental performance.

Eating after Training

If there are less than eight hours before the next training session, players should consume carbohydrate as soon as possible after the first session. This may then be followed by a meal a little later, or a series of small snacks, whichever a player finds most comfortable and practical. Carbohydrate requirement in this situation is at the rate of 1.0–1.2g per kg bodyweight per hour. When there is a longer period between training sessions, the pattern and timing of refuelling does not seem to be so critical. It is therefore up to the player how they organize their refuelling to fit in with other commitments. Carbohydrate-rich foods with moderate to high GI provide a readily available source of carbohydrate for resynthesis of muscle glycogen. Additional foods need to be included to provide protein and other nutrients, including anti-oxidants.

Suitable Pre-Training Meals and Snacks

Three to four hours before training:
- Toast, crumpets or bagels with jam or honey and a milk shake.
- Baked beans on toast.
- Cereal with banana and low fat milk.
- Sandwiches, rolls or baguettes with low fat spread and chicken, lean ham or tuna.
- Pasta or rice with a tomato sauce and very lean meat.

One to two hours before training:
- Milk shake or smoothie.
- Cereal bar or energy bar.
- Cereal with low fat milk.
- Low fat yogurt or rice.
- Fruit.

Less than one hour before training:
- Sports drink.
- Sports gel plus water.
- Sports bar.
- Jelly beans, jelly babies or M&S Percy Pigs.

Post-Exercise Meal Ideas

- French sticks, bagels or sandwiches made with white bread, fillings of tuna, salmon, chicken, lean meat and salad vegetables.
- White rice with stir-fry chicken and vegetables.
- Jacket potatoes with tuna and sweetcorn and salad.
- Breakfast cereal (not muesli or porridge) with low fat milk and banana.

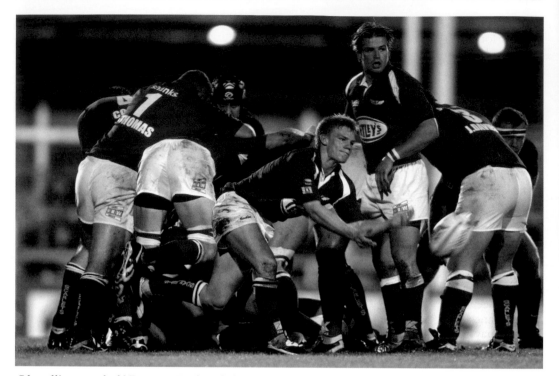

Llanelli scrum half Dwayne Peel feeds his back during the Heineken Cup Pool 3 match with Toulouse at Stradey Park, Llanelli in 2004. (© PA Photos)

Some players may find it hard to refuel through fatigue or loss of appetite. On the other hand, there may be poor access to food at the training venue. De-briefing sessions or treatment by the physio may delay the nutritional recovery process, too. Where lack of suitable food is the problem, players must take up this responsibility and have supplies in their kit bag or car. Consuming a sports drink during de-briefing or treatment will begin the process, and this should be followed by something more substantial at the first opportunity.

Eating Late and Sleep Patterns

It is a myth that eating close to bedtime should be avoided. It is also a myth that it leads to weight gain (as fat, not muscle). Eating a high carbohydrate meal will put fuel back into the muscles, not into the fat cells. Of course a daily intake greater than the body needs, regardless of meal timings, will lead to an increase in body fat and bodyweight. At

some time before bed, it is a good idea to think about what has been eaten during the day and spot if anything is missing. How much fruit has been eaten? How much milk, yogurt and cheese? Was carbohydrate intake sufficient? If not, then any gaps can be plugged before bed by having a banana or some dried fruit, a glass of milk or a couple of rounds of toast and honey. Nobody should go to bed feeling hungry.

Another reason often put forward for not eating late at night is that it could upset sleep patterns. If food and/or drink is the cause, it is invariably due to excessive intakes of alcohol, probably topped off with inappropriate high fat, fast foods such as doner kebabs (one of the greatest risks of food poisoning). None of the above suggestions, however, should cause sleep problems – in fact in most situations they could actually help a player get to sleep and have a quality night's sleep.

Sleep is a very important part of the recovery process, and research has shown that those whose lifestyle includes a high level of physical activity usually sleep more deeply and for longer than those who are less active. During sleep, all but the essential functions cease, and instead physiological repair and (if applicable) growth take place. These events peak during periods of deep sleep. There are several practical ways to ensure quality sleep. Going to bed at the same time each night helps the body to feel drowsy naturally; as a result there should be less difficulty getting to sleep than if bedtime is variable. An optimal environment for sleep is one that is quiet, dark, cool (ideally 18°C/65°F) and comfortable. A big bed is better than a narrow one as there can be forty to sixty position movements in the night, and having enough room to turn over is obviously important.

Mild sleep deprivation of one night of almost total sleeplessness before a match actually seems to have little effect on physical performance, but those who do worry that nerves may disrupt sleep patterns the night before an important match should try to get a few early nights in the week leading up to the match. Making the last meal before bed a high carbohydrate meal helps to increase the body's production of the hormone serotonin, which induces sleep. There is therefore some truth in the old wives' tale that a milky drink sweetened with honey encourages sleep. Having camomile tea at bedtime instead of regular tea or coffee, and sprinkling a little lavender on the pillow or a tissue placed on the pillow may also have a soporific effect – although some players may not feel comfortable doing the latter, especially if sharing a room.

Sleeping in a noisy environment or sharing a room with a snorer can usually be overcome with the use of ear plugs. Many élite sportspeople travel with their own pillow and a pile of relaxation DVDs such as dolphin sounds. On the other hand, counting sheep, watching violent or noisy films on TV or DVDs or listening to loud music with headphones should all be avoided; in other words, anything that stimulates the brain should be avoided.

CHAPTER 3

Fluids

Players need to keep their bodies well hydrated for their health and well-being, but also to maintain performance in training and matches. This can be achieved by drinking enough fluids to match ongoing losses from the body on a daily basis. If insufficient or inappropriate fluids are drunk, fluid balance will be compromised and this will certainly have a negative effect on performance, and in cases of severe dehydration, on health, too.

Daily Water Balance			
The following table monitors the daily water balance in a sedentary individual with a body mass of about 70–75kg living in a temperate climate. (*See* References Chapter 3, 1)			
Daily water input		*Daily water losses*	
Food	1,000ml	Urine	1,250ml
Drinks	1,200ml	Faeces	100ml
Metabolism	350ml	Skin	850ml
		Lungs	350ml
Total	2,550ml	*Total*	2,550ml

THE ROLE OF WATER IN THE BODY

Water has a key role in keeping the body alive. It is possible to survive for weeks without food, but the human body cannot survive more than a few days without water. In adults, water makes up 50 to 60 per cent of the total bodyweight. Water is an essential part of all the cells in the body as well as a major constituent of all bodily fluids such as blood, lymph and sweat; approximately 60 per cent of the body's water is inside the body cells (intracellular) and the remainder is outside (extracellular). Muscle contains about 75 per cent water by weight, whereas adipose tissue or body fat only contains 5 per cent. Women have larger stores of body fat and therefore less body water than men. It should come as no surprise that water is involved in a wide array of bodily functions:

- the transport of nutrients and oxygen;
- elimination of waste by the kidneys in urine;
- temperature regulation by the sweat-mechanism;
- swallowing (saliva);
- digestion (digestive juices);
- movement of joints and eyes, as a lubricant;
- transport of sound;
- maintenance of blood volume and blood pressure;
- respiration.

THE SWEAT MECHANISM

Muscles in active exercise produce heat, and a mechanism is needed to remove this excess heat from the body if the body temperature is to be kept within safe limits. Although a range of skin temperatures can be tolerated, the body's core temperature – or the temperature of the brain, heart, lungs and kidneys – must be kept constant: between 37° and 38°C. Increased heat production soon overloads the body's normal heat loss routes of conduction, convection and radiation, and to counter this shortfall the skin then employs two to four million heat-activated sweat glands, which can be recruited within seconds in response to the need to get rid of excessive amounts of heat. The sweat glands open up, leading to a secretion of sweat on to the surface of the skin: it is the evaporation of the sweat from the skin that actually cools the

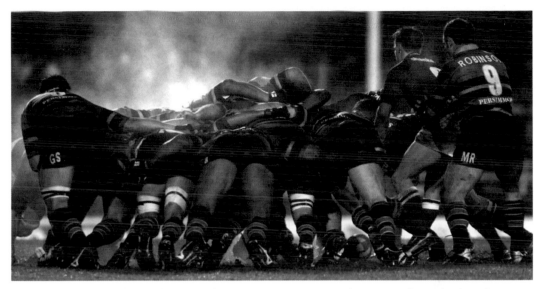

Llanelli Scarlets and Northampton Saints give off steam as they scrum down during the Heineken European Cup at Stradey Park, Llanelli in 2003. (© PA Photos)

body down, and this process can account for 80 per cent of heat lost during exercise.

Position Stand

In 2007 a *Position Stand* was published by the American College of Sports Medicine, which provides guidance on fluid replacement to help those people who are performing physical activity maintain appropriate hydration. (*See* References Chapter 3, 2.) It summarizes current knowledge on fluids and exercise from both the exercise performance and health points of view.

This *Position Stand* has replaced the previous one published in 1996. It provides a summary of current knowledge on exercise and fluid electrolyte needs, looks at the impact of fluid and electrolyte imbalances on exercise performance, as well as the impact of fluid and electrolyte imbalances on health. It also includes a *Strength of Recommendation Taxonomy* (SORT) to document the strength of evidence for each conclusion and recommendation made in the *Position Stand*.

Sweat Rates

The rate of sweating depends on a number of

ACMS Strength of Recommendation Taxonomy

A: Recommendation based on consistent and good quality experimental evidence (morbidity, mortality, exercise and cognitive performance, physiological responses).

B: Recommendation based on inconsistent or limited quality experimental evidence.

C: Recommendation based on consensus, usual practice, opinion, disease-oriented evidence,* case series or studies of diagnosis, treatment, prevention, or screening, or extrapolations from *quasi* experimental research.

* Patient-oriented evidence measures outcomes that matter to patients: morbidity, mortality, symptom improvement, cost reduction, and quality of life. Disease-oriented evidence measures intermediate, physiologic, or surrogate end points that may or may not reflect improvements in patient outcomes (for example blood pressure, blood chemistry, physiological function, pathological findings).

---

different factors. Thus the higher the intensity of a training session, the greater the heat production, and the higher the sweat rate will be. However, a longer training session at a lower intensity could produce greater overall sweat losses. Sweat rates in intermittent activity where exercise intensity keeps changing may be lower, because the breaks in activity allow heat production to diminish briefly. At constant exercise intensity, higher environmental temperatures lead to higher sweat rates, as does a higher humidity. During pre-season training in mid- to late summer players may train twice a day, and some players could carry a sweat loss from the first training session into the second one.

Improved fitness brings about a more efficient sweat response – as the body temperature rises during the training session, more sweat is lost sooner. This has the effect of cooling the body down, *but* it increases the need for players to be even more aware of their fluid requirements.

As the rugby season extends and becomes less of a truly winter sport, and the effects of global warming bring unseasonally warm days, teams should be aware of the impact that temperature and humidity can have on sweat rates. A sweat loss of 1.5ltr in a match played at 10–15°C could rise to 3.5–4.0ltr at 30–38°C. On humid days evaporation becomes less effective if the atmosphere is already laden with moisture, and instead sweat merely drips off the skin. This does not help in the cooling process, and the body reacts by producing even more sweat. On such days the risks of dehydration could be significant unless players realize the need to drink more.

As the cooling process is dependent on the evaporation of sweat from the skin, and not just its production, players should ensure that there is sufficient skin exposed to allow evaporation to take place. American footballers are almost completely covered with protective clothing, and as a consequence are at very high risk of serious dehydration. The risk to rugby players is considerably less, but they should still ensure that plenty of skin is 'on show'.

Bodyweight, genetic predisposition, heat acclimatization and how metabolically efficient an individual player is at performing a specific exercise, all influence sweat rates for a given activity. The range of sweat rates and the total amounts of sweat lost will vary considerably between players. In matches, the sweat rates of players will vary depending on their position and how long they are on the pitch.

ACMS Evidence Statement

Exercise can elicit high sweat rates and substantial water and electrolyte losses during sustained exercise, particularly in warm/hot weather. *Evidence Category A.*

There is considerable variability for water and electrolyte losses between individuals, and between different activities. *Evidence Category A.*

If sweat water and electrolyte losses are not replaced, then the person will dehydrate. *Evidence Category A.*

THE EFFECTS OF DEHYDRATION

If fluids are not replaced and the body becomes dehydrated, not only is performance impaired but health can also be put at risk. The plasma volume (the fluid component of blood) is needed to take oxygen and fuel to the working muscles, remove waste products, and of course to carry heat to the skin for removal. If sweat losses are not replaced the plasma volume drops, and this causes the heart rate to increase in order to keep up the cardiac output (the amount of blood pumped out with each heartbeat). Blood flow to the exercising muscles takes priority, so blood flow to the skin is reduced, sweat rate drops, and body temperature rises. This not only affects performance, but if unchecked when exercising on a particularly and unusually hot day, it can lead to fatigue.

A loss of body water corresponding to 2 per cent of bodyweight will start to impair performance and lead to premature tiredness. Perception of effort is increased for the same workload, and either a player will actually feel tired or, without realizing it, they will reduce their self-selected pace. However, other people will notice! These effects occur at all levels of dehydration, and increase as the degree of dehydration increases. Dehydration reduces mental functioning too, including decision-making, reaction times, concentration, anticipation, skill delivery and task accuracy.

Minimizing dehydration in matches could be the difference between winning – by scoring a try in the dying moments – and losing, by missing a crucial try-stopping tackle in those same dying moments. At this point it should come as no surprise that dehydration cannot be tolerated, largely because the body does not get used to dehydration.

Why Players Don't Drink Enough

There is no shortage of excuses given by people when asked why they are not drinking during exercise. Thirst is not a good indicator of dehydration, so waiting to feel thirsty is leaving it too late, as the body is already some way down the dehydration road. If fluids are not provided or available at the club, it is the players' responsibility to take their own drink and drinks bottle with them. Unlike other team sports, there are plenty of opportunities for players to drink during stoppages for injuries or goal kicks. Coaches should allow breaks during training sessions too, the frequency of these determined by the weather conditions and the intensity of the session.

The flavour, taste, mouth-feel and temperature of drinks can all affect how much is drunk. However, with such a wide range of drinks available every player should be able to find a suitable drink that they can stomach in both training and match situations. Some players worry about the gastro-intestinal consequences of drinking, particularly during intense training sessions as well as matches. This highlights the need to use lighter sessions to get used to the sensation of drinking, building up intake gradually and developing individual strategies of what, when and how much to drink. Interestingly nausea can actually be caused by dehydration itself.

The 'call of nature' is another excuse

> ### ACMS Evidence Statement
>
> Dehydration increases physiological strain and perceived effort to perform the same exercise task, and this is accentuated in warm/hot weather. *Evidence Category A.*
>
> Dehydration (> 2 per cent BW) can degrade aerobic exercise performance, especially in warm/hot weather. *Evidence Category A.*
>
> The greater the dehydration level, the greater the physiological strain and aerobic exercise performance decrement. *Evidence Category B.*
>
> Dehydration (> 2 per cent BW) might degrade mental/cognitive performance. *Evidence Category B.*
>
> Dehydration (3 per cent BW) has marginal influence on degrading aerobic exercise performance when cold stress is present. *Evidence Category B.*
>
> Dehydration (3–5 per cent BW) does not degrade either anaerobic performance or muscular strength. *Evidence Categories A and B.*
>
> The critical water deficit and the magnitude of exercise performance degradation are related to the heat stress, exercise task, and the individual's unique biological characteristics. *Evidence Category C.*
>
> Hyperhydration agents can be achieved by several methods, but provide equivocal benefits and have several disadvantages. *Evidence Category B.*

often given for poor fluid intake, in that the player is afraid of needing to urinate during a match and so doesn't drink enough beforehand. The secret is to get the timing right. Players should pass urine just before starting a match or training session in the knowledge that once they start exercising, urine production is drastically reduced as attention is directed towards the exercising muscles and away from urinary function.

WATER AND ELECTROLYTE LOSSES

Rugby is a team sport but played by individuals. This individuality becomes very apparent when looking at the sweat losses of players taking part in the same training sessions and playing in the same matches. Monitoring individual fluid and electrolyte losses can determine individual requirements, which can then be addressed in the training and match situations. It is useful to monitor bodyweight by weighing nude on reliable scales, first thing in the morning (after a visit to the loo); this will provide a baseline from which to measure dehydration. Players who are well hydrated and in energy balance will have a stable bodyweight that fluctuates by less than 1 per cent. Therefore a sudden loss of more than 0.5kg one morning could indicate a fluid shortfall in the previous day's fluid intake, assuming that a weight loss programme is not also being followed.

Measuring urine concentration as well as the early morning bodyweight can help to detect changes in fluid balance. However, measuring urine specific gravity (USG) and osmolality (UOsmol) are techniques that are unlikely to be available except to elite squads.

Sweat rates can be calculated by changes in bodyweight before and after training sessions, with appropriate corrections for the fluid intake during the particular session. Electrolytes, particularly salt or sodium, are lost regularly from the body in urine, faeces and sweat, and infrequently in some cases through vomiting. Measuring electrolyte losses will not be possible for most teams and players, but heavy salt sweaters can be identified in a number of quite simple ways. Such a player may complain of a very salty taste of sweat in the mouth, that the eyes become irritated when sweat gets into them, and – most noticeably – salt stains are visible on kit or skin: this shows as white marks on dark kit, particularly around the armpit and groin areas, and often as a white crustiness on the skin. Players who regularly have problems with muscle cramps could also be the same players who lose large amounts of salt in their sweat – though this is not always the case.

Little published data is available about sweat losses in rugby players, although individual international squads and clubs may well have data about their own players. The Department of Sports Nutrition at the Australian Institute of Sport (AIS) provides the following data on their website (www.ais.org.au/nutrition):

The following statistics are the mean fluid losses for male rugby union players under varying conditions:

Players	Sweat rate (litre/hour)	Ambient temperature (°C)	Relative humidity (%)
*	2.2	18–20	18–20
*	1.7	21–23	78–85
*	2.2	20–22	74–82
Forwards	2.6	24–25	30–32
Backs	1.6	24–25	30–32

* Position not specified.

Practical Advice

Weighing players before and after training can give a very rough indication of their level of dehydration. This takes account of the sweat loss and the amount of fluid consumed, and gives a net balance. More useful information can be obtained by weighing players and drinks bottles before and after training. The only equipment needed is a set of kitchen scales to weigh the bottles (in g) and a reliable set of scales to weigh the players (in kg) – although a little effort, organization and willingness on the part of the coaching, support staff and, of course, the players is essential too.

The information gathered can be put to good use. It identifies those players at most risk of becoming dehydrated so that strategies can be put in place to ensure that they have access to sufficient fluids in both training and match situations. For all players, but particularly young players, it can be a valuable educational tool. However, it must be remembered that there are errors in estimating hydration status by changes in bodyweight. However, it is the 'only realistic proxy measure of hypohydration for the

---

Determining Fluid Losses

The following is the protocol to determine individual fluid losses during training sessions:

- Record the weather conditions or the indoor temperature, depending on the training venue.
- Record pre-training bodyweight before warm-up starts, after the last visit to the loo, naked or with minimal clothing (underpants), and bare-footed.
- Record post-training bodyweight (less than 10min after training finishes) after towel drying and naked, or with clean, dry underpants and bare-footed. (Note: sweaty underpants can distort the results considerably.)
- Label drinks bottles to reduce the risk of players using the wrong bottle.
- Players must be clear that they can only drink from their own bottle.
- Fluids must not be spat out or poured over the head.
- All drinks bottles should be weighed empty, and then again full with the appropriate fluid.
- If drinks bottles need to be refilled they must be re-weighed.
- Drinks bottles should be weighed at the same time as the final bodyweight is measured.

Sweat loss (litres) = bodyweight before exercise (kg) − bodyweight after exercise (kg) + fluid consumed during exercise (litres).

Sweat loss can be converted to a sweat rate per hour by dividing the sweat loss by the exercise time in minutes and multiplying by sixty.

---

and urine colour darkens, so the volume and frequency of urinating both decrease, too. Monitoring urinating habits yourself is a non-invasive, inexpensive and immediate way of evaluating hydration status. However, urine colour can be influenced by factors that are not related to hydration status, such as diet (eating beetroot, for example), medication (and particularly the regular use of vitamin supplements containing the vitamin B2 or riboflavin) and illness.

For those players wishing to take up this easy method of self-monitoring, laminated credit-card-sized pee charts and A4 posters can be bought from Dietitians in Sport and Exercise Nutrition (*see* Appendix VI for the address). The chart gives six graded colours, from very pale – almost colourless – to a rich brown colour. In some situations players will be able to have their first morning urine samples measured for specific gravity (USG) and urine osmolality (UOsmol); however, for the vast majority of players this will not be an option.

DIETARY FACTORS

Players should not forget the major contribution the diet makes in terms of fluid intake, and in ensuring a normal body-water content

athlete and the field-based practitioner'. (*See* References Chapter 3, 3.)

Hydration Indicators in Urine

Changes in urine colour, specific gravity (measure of the density of urine compared to water) and osmolality (concentration) occur with increasing degrees of dehydration. The colour darkens, and specific gravity and osmolality increase as the kidneys try to conserve fluid losses. As dehydration develops

---

ACMS Evidence Statement

Individuals can monitor their hydration status by employing simple urine and bodyweight measurements. *Evidence Category B.*

An individual with a 'first morning' USG < 1.020 or UOsmol < 700mOsmol/kg can be considered as euhydrated. *Evidence Category B.*

Several days of 'first morning' bodyweights can be used to establish baseline bodyweights that represent euhydration. *Evidence Category B.*

Bodyweight changes can reflect sweat losses during exercise, and can be used to calculate individual fluid replacement needs for specific exercise and environmental conditions. *Evidence Category A.*

Water Content of Selected Foods			
(Measured in grams per 100g edible portion)			
Bananas	76g	Melon	92g
Butter,	16g	Low fat spread	50g
margarine		Milk	88g
Cheese	36g	Potatoes	79g
Chips	57g	Chicken	75g
Eggs	75g	Lettuce	95g
Oranges	86g	White fish	82g
Yogurt	77g	Peanuts	6g
Crisps	2g		
(1g equivalent to 1ml)			

(euhydration), not just as drinks but food as well.

The electrolyte losses in sweat, particularly sodium and potassium, must be replenished, and players will easily replace these by the food they eat after training and matches. People are often advised by pseudo-nutritionists and journalists to avoid coffee because of the dehydrating effects of caffeine, particularly in situations where fluid balance may be compromised. However, a review published in 2003 looked at the current literature concerning the effect of caffeine ingestion on fluid balance (*see* References Chapter 3, 4), and concluded that there was no support for the suggestion that consumption of caffeine-containing beverages as part of a normal lifestyle led to fluid loss in excess of

---

ACSM Evidence Statement

Meal consumption promotes euhydration. *Evidence Category A.*

Sweat electrolyte (sodium and potassium) losses should be fully replaced to establish euhydration. *Evidence Category A.*

Caffeine consumption will not markedly alter daily urine output or hydration status. *Evidence Category B.*

Alcohol consumption can increase urine output and delay full rehydration. *Evidence Category B.*

---

the volume ingested (that is, that it has a diuretic effect).

Caffeine consumption was not associated with poor hydration status, either. Players who habitually drink caffeine-containing drinks can be reassured that intakes of less than 300mg of caffeine a day will not compromise hydration status (this is roughly equivalent to three mugs of coffee or six cups of tea). Alcohol, on the other hand, does act as a diuretic, especially in high doses, and consumption should therefore be moderate, particularly in the initial period after training and matches.

FLUID INTAKE AND THE TRAINING REGIME

Fluid Intake before Exercise

A player should begin training or matches with a normal body-water content (he/she should be euhydrated). If regular meals have been taken, and plenty of fluids, and there has been sufficient recovery time since the last training session, the player should be suitably hydrated. However, this may not apply to the élite player who does more than one training session in a day. During pre-season training when the weather conditions alone may be causing an increased sweat rate, players will need to pay specific attention to their fluid intake so they do not start any training sessions dehydrated. Players should aim to consume 5–7ml per kg bodyweight at least four hours before training. If urine is dark or none is passed, a player should drink

---

ACMS Recommendations

Prehydrating with beverages, if needed, should be initiated at least several hours before the exercise task to enable fluid absorption and allow urine output to return towards normal levels. Consuming beverages with sodium and/or salted snacks or small meals with beverages can help to stimulate thirst and retain needed fluids.

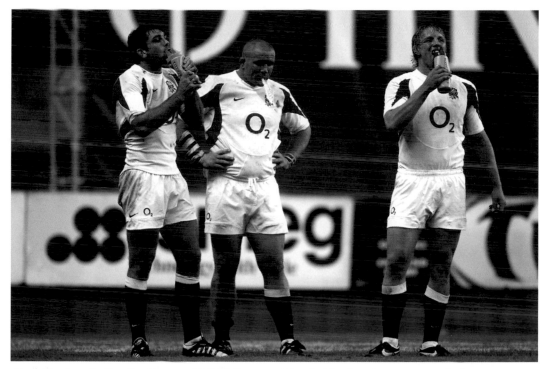

(l–r) England's Pat Sanderson, Phil Vickery and Lewis Moody take on some refreshments. (© PA Photos)

more about two hours before training starts. This time the amount should be around 3–5ml per kg bodyweight. Consuming fluids ahead of training allows enough time for urine output to return to normal before the start of training. Fluids that contain sodium (sports drinks), and salty snacks or food, can help to drive the thirst mechanism as well as help the body retain the fluid.

Fluid Intakes during Exercise

Players should aim to prevent fluid losses greater than 2 per cent of bodyweight. The amount and rate of fluid intake during exercise will depend on individual sweat rates, the duration of the training session, and what opportunities coaches offer to drink. Players should monitor bodyweight changes during different types and durations of training and in different weather conditions. Keeping this information, together with a record of approximate fluid intake during the session, in a training log can be an invaluable tool allowing players to develop their own hydration strategies.

ACMS Recommendations

Individuals should develop customized fluid replacement programmes that prevent excessive (< 2 per cent bodyweight reductions from baseline bodyweight) dehydration. The routine measurement of pre- and post-exercise bodyweights is useful for determining sweat rates and customized fluid replacement programmes. Consumption of beverages containing electrolytes and carbohydrates can help sustain fluid-electrolyte balance and exercise performance.

Fluid Intakes after Exercise

However hard a player has worked at the fluid intake before and during training or a match, they will probably still need to replace variable amounts of fluid and electrolytes after training. The only exception is likely to be a training session of short duration and very light intensity on a cool day. Sports drinks offer a very convenient way to replace fluids and electrolytes and to start the restocking of carbohydrate stores in the muscles.

In many situations, a meal with some added salt and water to drink will be quite enough to replace fluids, electrolytes and carbohydrate – if consumed in sufficient amounts. Players undertaking more than one training session in a day, and therefore needing to recover rapidly, should drink up to 1.5ltr of a sports drink for every kilogram of weight loss.

ACMS Recommendations

If time permits, consumption of normal meals and beverages will restore euhydration. Individuals needing rapid and complete recovery from excessive dehydration can drink 1.5ltr of fluid for each kilogram of bodyweight lost. Consuming beverages and snacks with sodium will help to expedite rapid and complete recovery by stimulating thirst and fluid retention. Intravenous fluid replacement is generally not advantageous, unless medically merited.

Match Strategies

Having established in training sessions which players in the squad are likely to lose the greatest percentage of fluid on a bodyweight basis, a match strategy can be developed. This should ensure that all players have opportunities to take on board fluids, but that those at greatest risk of dehydration are specifically targeted when stoppages in play allow.

When possible, replacements and, of course, physiotherapists should take every opportunity to go on to the pitch with water bottles. They may need to be prompted to do this by members of the coaching or medical staff present. Bottles could also be placed behind the goal-posts if this is feasible. Again, if it is practical, bottles could be made available on the opposite side to the bench, with

a non-player available to supervise the distribution of the bottles and ensure that refilled bottles are available for the second half, too.

If there are any 'special' drinks it would make sense for one person to be responsible for them. It is important that the player taking goal kicks is not forgotten, but is also given the opportunity to have a drink. Offering fluids to the referee might also be considered a wise move, too.

The opportunity to drink during half-time (and to pee) should be taken, particularly by those players who struggle to drink during the actual match. The same strategies should be employed for away matches and when playing abroad.

Fluid Intake and Team Management

Players will need encouragement and help if they are to meet the guidelines already discussed. Coaches or team management should ensure that suitable fluids and bottles are made available at training and matches, or that players bring their own, equally suitable drinks and bottles. They should schedule drinks breaks into training sessions and remind players to take these opportunities to drink, particularly those identified to be at greatest risk of dehydration.

An educational session on hydration should be organized during pre-season training.

Sweat loss and fluid intake monitoring should be carried out at intervals (but not too frequently that it becomes a chore for everybody) to help players recognize their individual losses in different training and weather conditions. On the basis of this data strategies should be devised to target players at most risk of dehydration during matches, with fluids at every feasible opportunity.

SPORTS DRINKS

When players drink in the training and match situations they want the fluids to be digested and absorbed as quickly as possible. Depending on the choice of drink, stomach emptying may be slowed up, as may absorption across the wall of the small intestine. If this happens there will be a delay in getting fluid into the circulation and carbohydrate into the fatiguing muscles. A number of factors affect the rate of stomach emptying:

- Volume — High volume speeds up emptying.
- Fat — High fat content slows down emptying.
- Osmolality — Hypertonic solutions slow emptying (they are more concentrated).
- pH — Low pH (more acidic) slows emptying.
- Calorie density — High calorie density slows emptying.
- Carbohydrate concentration — > 8 per cent slows empyting.
- Carbohydrate type — No effect.
- Exercise type — No effect.
- Exercise level — 0–70 per cent VO_{2max} no effect. > 75 per cent VO_{2max} slows emptying.
- Dehydration — Slows emptying during exercise.

Once the drink reaches the small intestine, the presence of glucose and sodium actually increases the rate of water absorption compared to plain water. Other carbohydrates, such as sucrose or glucose polymers, can be substituted for glucose without impairing glucose or water uptake. Lucozade Sport, Powerade and Taut Endurance are examples of sports drinks.

Home-Made Sports Drinks

Some players may have suitable sports drinks provided for them by their club. For those players who do not get supplies bought for them, buying enough drinks to meet fluid requirements can become quite expensive. A cheaper, though perhaps less convenient, way of ensuring that the correct fluid is being drunk is to make up a sports drink.

Toothcare

Dentists have two major problems with the

Recipes for Home-made Sports Drinks

Recipe 1
500ml unsweetened fruit juice (e.g. orange, pineapple or grapefruit)
500ml water
1 large pinch of salt (1.0–1.5g or ⅕ teaspoon)
Dissolve the salt in a little of the water, which has been warmed. Add the fruit juice and remaining water (not warmed). Mix together, cover, and keep chilled in the fridge.

Recipe 2
200ml squash (any flavour, but *not* low sugar/no added sugar varieties)
Make up to 1ltr with water
1 large pinch of salt (1.0–1.5g or ⅕ teaspoon)
Dissolve the salt in a little warm water. Add the squash, and then make up to 1ltr with cool water. Mix together, cover and keep chilled in the fridge.

Recipe 3
50–70g glucose or sucrose (ordinary sugar)
1ltr warm water
1 large pinch of salt (1.0–1.5g or ⅕ teaspoon)
Dissolve the sugar and salt in the water. Allow to cool, cover, and keep chilled in the fridge. Flavour with low sugar or low calorie squash (not regular, as this will upset the balance of carbohydrate) and then top up to 1ltr with water.

Make up a new batch of drink every day. Throw away any unused drink after twenty-four hours. Keep water bottles very clean, as sugary drinks attract bugs and other nasty things: this is important at all times, but especially during warmer weather.

use of sports drinks: dental decay and dental erosion. Dental decay is caused by dental plaque, a thin layer of bacteria that sticks to the teeth and breaks down sugars in the diet into acids, which in turn attack the teeth. Anything that contains sugars will have the ability to contribute to dental decay.

Dental erosion is a different problem and does not involve bacteria. It occurs when acids from the diet or regurgitated from the stomach, as happens if a player vomits, dissolve the tooth surface. The main sources of acid in the diet are fruits, particularly citrus fruits such as oranges, grapefruits and lemons, fruit juices, fruit-based and fizzy soft drinks, pickled foods or foods containing vinegar and sports drinks.

Most dentists accept that it is vital for players to keep well hydrated, and that sports drinks play an important part in achieving good hydration status. Sports drinks should therefore not be avoided because of the risk of development of dental erosion: instead, great care should be taken to ensure that the risks of erosion and decay are minimized as much as possible.

Care of Bottles

Great care should be taken to keep drinks bottles scrupulously clean, particularly if a sports drink is used. The carbohydrate in the drink makes them particularly attractive to fast-growing bacteria that will happily multiply at a great rate. Even if players have only used water, similar precautions should be taken, particularly if bottles are thrown around muddy pitches (as they frequently are).

Bottles should be washed thoroughly every time they have been used. Hot, soapy water must be used, and the bottle should be left to air-dry rather than be dried with a tea-towel. Bottles should be stored without their lids on, too. Once or twice a week it is advisable to sterilize bottles with a baby-bottle sterilizing fluid or denture-sterilizing tablets, whichever is to hand!

Energy Drinks

Since caffeine is no longer on the WADA Prohibited List (though it is still included in the Monitoring Programme, in competition only), use of energy drinks has become popular in some sports, including rugby. It must be understood that these drinks should not be used when fluid replacement is the goal. The high carbohydrate content and lack of sodium in most products could actually slow up the hydrating process. Therefore in situations where dehydration could have a negative impact on performance, they should not

Guidelines to Minimize Dental Problems

- Sports drinks should be drunk quickly, avoiding any sipping, holding or swishing of the fluid in the mouth.
- Try to squirt the drink behind the teeth and swallow quickly so the drink does not have any contact with the teeth. Take care to avoid choking, though.
- Where possible, cool drinks should be used as this can help to reduce the erosion. However, with a team sport this is not always possible.
- Mouth guards should never be rinsed with a sports drink, only with water.
- For at least an hour after using a sports drink, or any other acidic drink or food, tooth-brushing should be avoided. A mouthwash can be used instead.
- Sports drinks should only be used before, during and after matches and appropriate training sessions (where sweat losses are expected to be quite high). Intake of other acidic drinks during the day should be monitored and limited if necessary.
- Sugar-free chewing gum is tooth friendly. It helps to clear away food debris and increase saliva production. Saliva is alkaline in nature and so helps to neutralize the acid. Gum should only be used immediately *after* training or matches when a sports drink has been used. Chewing gum during exercise is a very bad idea because of the risk of choking.
- Have fruit juice at meal times when the food will stimulate saliva flow and so neutralize the acid.
- Once teeth have been cleaned at bedtime, nothing more should be eaten or drunk apart from water. This is because the flow of saliva falls during sleep.
- Flossing and brushing with de-sensitizing fluoride toothpaste should be undertaken twice a day.
- Regular check-ups with a dentist and hygienist will indicate whether enough care is being taken of the teeth.

be integrated into a player's existing hydration strategy. In terms of the other ingredients in the most popular energy drinks, caffeine would appear to be the only one with proven value, as will be discussed in Chapter 7. These drinks should give a measured dose of caffeine as declared on the can.

Sports Waters

Sports waters are hypotonic drinks with a much lower carbohydrate content and a lighter flavour than sports drinks. The inclusion of sodium and flavouring may improve overall fluid intake in people who normally drink only water. Their lower carbohydrate and energy content makes them a drink more suitable for low intensity exercise, particularly in cooler weather conditions when sweat losses will be low. They are not the best choice when rapid rehydration is necessary, for instance in warm/hot weather or when the supply of energy is vital.

It is unlikely that players will choose a sports water, as in most situations a sports drink will be far more beneficial in terms of replacing sweat losses and topping up flagging energy sources; otherwise they will probably just drink plain tap or bottled water. Examples of sports waters include Lucozade Sport Hydro Active and Aqua.

Oxygenated Water

It has been claimed that drinking oxygenated water during exercise could have a beneficial, even truly ergogenic effect on performance. In other words, 'drinking' oxygen would supplement the oxygen that was being breathed in. Presumably the designers of such drinks had noticed that people tend to breathe harder as exercise intensity increases. In fact tiny amounts of oxygen can be dissolved in drinking water, though this is a mere drop in the ocean compared to the amount of oxygen needed for exercise. Of course the oxygen has to be absorbed into the body from the intestine, but unlike the lung this particular part of the body is not designed to absorb gas. Analysis of these waters has shown that a breath of fresh air contains more O_2 than a litre of hyperoxygenated water. In a leader article in the *British Journal of Sports Medicine*, the author concluded that 'ergogenic claims for oxygenated water cannot be taken seriously'. (*See* References Chapter 3, 5.)

Permission to reproduce sections of the American College of Sports Medicine Position Stand 'Exercise and Fluid replacement' (*Medicine and Science in Sports and Exercise*, 39 (2), 277–390) has been obtained from Lippincott Williams and Wilkins, Baltimore, USA.

CHAPTER 4
Matches and Tournaments

Home and away matches are played in weekly leagues throughout the season. In addition there can be cup matches which may involve matches abroad. Included in the fixture list for some players will be tournaments with several games played in a single day, as happens in a sevens competition. In the case of the World Cup, matches are played over several weeks, invariably in a foreign country for the majority of players.

Most work periods for all players are less than 4sec in duration and rarely continue for more than 15sec. (*See* References Chapter 4, 1.) High intensity periods can follow each other leading to dense phases of play. Average rest periods during matches are often overstated by the other breaks in play that take place during stoppages for injuries and time out for penalty goals and conversions. Rest periods are usually 0 to 20sec, though rest periods of over 100sec can be 'enjoyed' by some of the backs. Players need to maintain their performance for as long as they are on the pitch, which could be for the entire match, until they are substituted, or are unlucky enough to be forced to retire to the bench or treatment room through injury. Enforced rest periods of 10min can also occur through sin-binning.

Depleted stores of fuel can be a potential problem for players on the pitch for the entire match, particularly if they have not made the necessary pre-match dietary preparations. Similarly, not starting the match well hydrated, and/or ignoring the opportunities to take on board fluids during the match and at half-time, can also reflect in a decline in performance. Good match nutrition not only helps physical performance towards the end of the match, but it can also help to maintain skills and judgement until the final whistle. It

may indeed make the difference between winning and losing. In a contact sport like rugby, injuries obviously happen for a whole variety of different reasons, many of which cannot be controlled. However, players can at least reduce the risk of picking up an injury through fatigue by going into every match well prepared.

Nutritional Match Goals

Players should ensure they
- start with sufficient supplies of energy to minimize fatigue and tired muscles towards the end of the match in order to:
- start the match well hydrated;
- maintain good hydration throughout the match;
- start the match feeling comfortable internally.

PRE-MATCH PREPARATION

Depletion of carbohydrate or glycogen stores and dehydration are the major causes of early fatigue in matches. The aim of the pre-match meal is therefore to top up the fuel stores in muscles and in the liver. Topping up the liver stores is particularly important if the kick-off is in the morning when these stores will be depleted after the overnight fast. The pre-match meal can also help to calm down any hunger pangs while still leaving the stomach feeling settled and comfortable.

Maintenance of good hydration status in the run-up to the match is equally important. What is eaten and drunk pre-match can not only prepare the body physically, but it can also have a psychological impact, too. Knowing that the planned dietary and fluid preparation has been completed satisfactorily can give some peace of mind at a time of increased nervous tension. If the pre-match meal is eaten as a team this can also provide an opportunity to boost morale and talk about tactics, focus players, and of course ensure that all players are well fuelled and well hydrated.

Composition of Pre-Match Intake

The amount of carbohydrate consumed in the pre-match meal is important. Laboratory studies have shown that although small amounts of carbohydrate consumed pre-exercise improve endurance capacity, greater amounts are even more effective. However, in the non-laboratory situation intakes are likely to be much less, as consuming large amounts invariably leads to gastro-intestinal discomfort. Therefore a balance is obviously needed so that a player consumes enough carbohydrate to support performance, but not so much that they feel uncomfortable or uneasy.

The type of carbohydrate chosen can also have an impact on performance. Different types of carbohydrate produce quite different changes in blood glucose levels and insulin concentrations. This is the theory behind the classification into low, medium and high glycaemic index for different carbohydrate foods. This concept is explained in more depth in Chapter 2. Studies have shown that endurance capacity is improved after a low glycaemic index meal compared to after a high glycaemic index meal. (*See* References Chapter 4, 2.)

This effect seems to be caused by a greater rate of fat oxidation and more stable blood glucose concentrations. With the increase in fat oxidation there is a reduction in carbohydrate breakdown, and as a result the limited stores of muscle glycogen are spared. (*See* References Chapter 4, 2.) Williams and Serratosa suggest that consuming enough carbohydrate in pre-match meals is probably the most important strategy for football players because of the lack of opportunities to take on board carbohydrate during a football match. Although there are more stoppages and therefore more opportunities to drink sports drinks during rugby matches, many

---

Characteristics of High and Low GI Meals

(These characteristics are for a 70kg subject.)
(*See* References Chapter 4, 2.)

High-GI breakfast	*Providing*
72g Corn Flakes	852kcal
300ml skimmed milk	162g carbohydrate
93g white bread	12g fat
12g Flora spread	23g protein
23g jam	Glycaemic index 78
181ml Lucozade Original	

Low-GI breakfast	*Providing*
100g muesli	855kcal
(without raisins)	162g carbohydrate
300ml skimmed milk	11g fat
78g apple	27g protein
120g tinned peaches	Glycaemic index 44
149g yogurt	
300ml apple juice	

---

players do not use these opportunities, and many more do not drink a sports drink, preferring to drink only water. If players cannot be persuaded to drink sports drinks they should at least heed the advice to consume low GI foods in their pre-match meal. All players should be aware that consuming a high carbohydrate meal before the match, and a sports drink during the match, leads to a greater exercise capacity than the high carbohydrate meal alone.

Practical Advice

For most players their last meal should be about three hours before the kick-off. If the kick-off is at midday, the meal will be break-

---

Advantages of a Low GI Pre-Match Meal

- Long-term stable blood glucose concentrations.
- General feelings of satiety.
- Delayed onset of fatigue in muscles.
- Positive influences on the central nervous system and brain in particular, making the player feel better (often the basis of a good performance in itself).

fast; if the match starts in the late afternoon (around 3.00pm) the player should have a light breakfast followed by a lunch; and if it is an evening kick-off the player should have a late breakfast, a light lunch, and a pre-match meal between 3.00pm and 4.00pm.

The pre-match meal should, of course, be high in carbohydrate but with a low amount of fibre, particularly if a player regularly suffers from an over-active digestive system because of pre-match nerves. It should also be low in fat and contain low to moderate amounts of protein. The meal should not be too bulky or filling, nor should it be particularly salty and certainly not spicy. If the club is providing the food, a reasonable selection should be available so that all players can have something they enjoy and are familiar eating pre-match. A short questionnaire pre-season to all the playing squad to elicit pre-match likes and dislikes could be a very worthwhile exercise in terms of keeping catering costs down, avoiding wastage, and ensuring a suitably nourished team.

Some players who have eaten a meal three

Suitable Pre-Match Meals

- Low fibre breakfast cereal or porridge with low fat milk and sugar or syrup.
- Granary or multigrain bread or toast with low fat spread and jam, marmalade or honey.
- Pancakes with syrup or honey.
- Müller low fat yogurt or rice pudding.
- Low fat milk shakes, smoothies or meal replacements (such as Build-Up or Complan).
- Bananas.
- Cereal bars.
- Sandwiches or rolls (ideally granary bread) with low fat spread and chicken, lean ham, tuna or salmon fillings.
- Jacket potatoes with low fat toppings (baked beans, low fat soft cheese or tuna).
- Spaghetti in tomato sauce on toast (granary if possible).
- Baked beans on granary or pitta bread.
- Pasta and tomato sauce with/without small chicken breast.
- Noodles with chicken.

---

hours before the kick-off can start to feel a little peckish. If a sports drink (which all players would do well to use in the run-up to the start of the match) is not satisfying enough they could top up with a banana, some dried fruit, a few jelly beans, jelly babies or Marks and Spencer Percy Pigs. Back in the 1970s the results from one or two studies suggested that consuming carbohydrate in the hour before exercise would have a negative effect on performance: they showed that muscle glycogen was used up faster after a concentrated carbohydrate drink had been consumed and, as a consequence, fatigue set in sooner. However, many more subsequent studies have not been able to reproduce the results, and this advice seems to be no longer valid.

DURING THE MATCH

The main priority during a match is to drink appropriate fluids. Some players do eat jelly beans, jelly babies, bananas or Jaffa cakes at half-time and feel comfortable in the second half, but the majority of players will be content with taking on board just fluids. Certainly those players who eat very little or even nothing before a match will benefit from drinking a sports drink during the match and at half-time. Players who avoid sports drinks – which provide fluid, carbohydrate and electrolytes – in favour of water should experiment with these drinks during rugby training sessions. Once used to them in the training environment they should begin to use them in matches, too. The number of players who persist in using water rather than a sports drink in training and matches continues to surprise the author, since there is considerable evidence to show that, far from being a marketing 'con', using a sports drink can have a significant positive impact on performance. Some players may prefer to use a carbohydrate gel and water at half-time. The end result will be the same as if the players had drunk a sports drink, as long as they consume sufficient water with the gel.

Players on the bench have unlimited opportunities to take fluids on board, and in

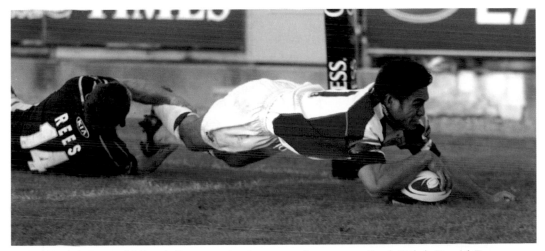

Bristol Rugby's David Lemi dives over in the corner for a try as Leeds Tyke's David Rees tackles him. (© PA Photos)

some cases an element of caution may be needed to prevent them drinking too much. For example, there may not always be sufficient notice to make a visit to the cloakroom before a player goes on to the pitch.

Unlike many other team sports, rugby provides an opportunity to take fluids on board not only at half-time, but during the match too. During stoppages, drinks can be taken on to the pitch by physiotherapists and a limited number of non-playing team members. The training environment provides an opportunity to identify those players most at risk of becoming dehydrated during matches: once this has been done, a match plan can be devised to target these players specifically during stoppages. This, together with the performance and health benefits of using sports drinks, is covered in detail in Chapter 3.

AFTER THE MATCH

Once the final whistle has blown it is important to rehydrate and refuel as soon as possible, exactly the same as after a hard training session. Fluid losses need to be replaced and carbohydrates consumed quickly. Glycogen stores are replaced quickest in the 15 to 30min immediately after the match finishes, and still at a faster-than-normal rate up to two hours after the match has finished. Some

Suitable Provisions for the Changing Room

Sports drinks are the best way to rehydrate and start replenishing depleted muscle glycogen stores. Otherwise the following provisions should be provided:

- Fresh fruit – including bananas.
- Dried fruit.
- Fruit juices.
- Smoothies or milkshakes.
- Sandwiches/rolls/bagels* with tuna, lean ham, chicken and salmon** fillings (i.e. good quality protein but low in fat).
- Thick-crust pizza slices with lean meat, vegetable toppings and a sprinkling of cheese (to keep fat intake low).
- Sports bars.
- Cereal bars. There are now so many to choose from and they all have similar nutritional values that it does not matter which ones are provided. It is probably best to ring the changes throughout the season so that players do not become bored.

* Both white and wholemeal bread have high glycaemic indexes compared to other types of bread, and are absorbed into the body quickly: they should therefore be the first choice.
** Salmon is slightly higher in fat content but it is 'good' fat, and it also has properties that can help the repair of tissues after a match.

protein should also be included, as it not only helps the storage of carbohydrate in the muscles but is also needed for the repair of muscle and tissue damage that will have occurred. Nor should vitamin and mineral intakes be forgotten: these nutrients are important because they are involved in the general repair of the body after strenuous exercise.

Ideally suitable food and fluids should be provided in the changing room for immediate consumption. Selection may be limited but it should provide enough choice to make sure there is something suitable for all players.

After making inroads into the food and drinks available in the changing room, players should be encouraged to eat a carbohydrate-rich, moderate protein and lowish fat meal in the early evening following an afternoon kick-off. In some situations this will be a meal provided at the ground. Adopting a team approach and providing a post-match meal helps to ensure that all players complete their refuelling and rehydrating quickly and therefore effectively.

Suitable light but nutritionally sound meals to have at home after an evening kick-off (if nothing is provided) include simple, quick meals such as baked beans on toast, or cereals with milk and a banana or dried fruit. The nutritional content should not only help recovery, but should also encourage a good night's sleep too – if any encouragement is needed after a hard match.

In some situations teams may have to play two matches in less than seven days, such as on a Sunday afternoon and then on the following Friday night. The Christmas and New Year holiday period can also see players undertaking two matches with little space between to recover. In these situations players need to make a concerted effort to ensure they consume enough carbohydrate to fully replace muscle glycogen stores between the matches.

According to a paper published in 2006, the nutritional practices of rugby league players in Australia were best in the lead-up to matches and worst in the period immediately after matches (see References Chapter 4, 3). The day after matches, energy intake was low, with less energy coming from carbohydrate and more energy provided from alcohol and fat than on other days – the carbohydrate intake was in fact about half the recommended intake.

The authors suggest that this may reflect the difficulty players have in consuming such large amounts of carbohydrate. Two other reasons put forward were that the players felt they needed to reward themselves after the match and the previous weeks of training, or they simply did not understand the importance of nutrition in recovery. Alcohol was generally consumed in substantial amounts in the immediate post-match period, with approximately a third of players having an intake above what is considered to be the safe level in Australia.

Post-Match Alcohol

After matches – and after training sessions, too, amongst the non-élite – alcohol can play an important part in team bonding and, unlike football, players can often enjoy mixing socially with the fans. Excessive intakes are not uncommon, but they can hinder post-match recovery and be counter-productive if a player is attempting to reduce body fat levels. However, by keeping to normal guidelines for the population, health and performance should not be impaired except perhaps by hindering post-exercise recovery. Players should refuel and rehydrate after matches before even considering consuming alcohol.

Eating Out Post-Match

Some players may well go out in a crowd after a match to celebrate or commiserate, but this is not a valid reason to avoid the initial refuelling and rehydrating in the changing room. Suitable meals can be chosen in most types of restaurant, although this may require an element of will-power when less appropriate items can look more appealing. The aim is to try to avoid eating too much fat, and to concentrate on carbohydrate-rich meals with good quality protein. In restaurants, if players are in any doubt about a particular dish, they should ask the waiter, but in

Examples of Restaurant Choices

The following are examples of good and not-so-good restaurant choices:

Chinese

Chinese meals tend to contain lots of vegetables and not much fat apart from the obvious deep-fried items. Most menus give descriptions of the ingredients in a dish and how it is cooked.

Good
Soup
Crispy duck
Stir-fries
Steamed dishes
Plain boiled rice
Noodles

Not So Good
Prawn crackers and spring rolls
Sweet and sour dishes
Spare ribs
Fried rice
If overeating is a potential problem, using chopsticks can usually slow down eating and reduce overall consumption.

Fast food
Good
Plain burger with lettuce, tomato and an extra bun
Milkshake

Not So Good
Chicken burger (deep-fried)
Cheese
Mayonnaise
French fries (thin, as they absorb more fat than thick ones)

French and Italian
Good
Bread and breadsticks
Minestrone soup
Grilled, steamed, poached, baked, casseroled or roasted meat, fish or poultry
Tomato-based sauces (Napoletana, Marinara, Bolognese)
Pasta, rice or boiled potatoes

Not so good
Garlic bread
Whitebait
Pesto
Carbonara
Dishes with creamy sauces
Fried, battered, creamed, buttered, sautéed or *au gratin* dishes

Greek

Greek meals are built around salad vegetables, bread, pasta, rice and a lot of olive oil. Olive oil is actually pretty healthy, but – like most things – not in excess.

Good
Tzatziki, houmous and pitta bread
Greek salad with feta cheese (a lower fat variety of cheese)
Grilled meats and fish
Kebabs
Stuffed peppers, tomatoes or vine leaves
Plain rice
Boiled potatoes
Greek yogurt and fruit

Not so good
Fried foods, such as calamari

Indian
Again, menus usually explain what each dish contains, and sometimes how it has been cooked.

Good
Soups – lentil (dahl)
Raita (cucumber or onion with yogurt)
Tandoori and tikka dishes
Kebabs
Biryanis, dhansak, rogan josh, jalfrezi
Plain rice, naan, chapattis, roti and paratha

Not so good
Samosas
Crispy rolls
Fried starters
Kormas, pasandas and masalas (all have creamy sauces)
Anything cooked in lots of ghee (clarified butter)
Special fried rice
Puris
All puddings

continued overleaf

Examples of Restaurant Choices *continued*

Mexican

Good

Enchiladas and burritos (but check the amount of cheese and cream)

Fajitas

Sour cream and guacamole, but only in small amounts

Rice

Not so good

Corn chips, deep-fried potato skins

Tostadas

Pizza

Good

Deep pan pizzas

Ham and pineapple pizza

Margherita pizza

Vegetarian pizza

Seafood pizza

Vegetable toppings

Not so good

Salami and pepperoni pizza

Extra cheese

Traditional pubs

Good

Jacket potatoes with baked beans, chilli or tuna

Shepherd's pie with vegetables

Ploughman's with more bread and less cheese

Soups with bread

Sandwiches

Not so good

Most savoury snacks

Anything fried

---

general should avoid anything described as pan-fried, buttered, creamed, fried or sautéed.

REFEREES

Referees need to follow similar advice to players with regard to diet and fluids for themselves for both training and matches if they are to minimize fatigue, particularly during matches. Practical issues involving hydration during matches need to be addressed, too. It might be possible to speak to support staff at the home ground to ensure that the referee's own water bottle is carried on to the pitch by non-playing players, or even the physiotherapist. Touch judges can keep a bottle on the side line for use at convenient moments.

Consuming a sports drink, particularly at half-time, will provide water and sodium to hydrate the body, and carbohydrate to delay the onset of fatigue and to minimize dehydration. Not only does dehydration affect physical performance, it also has an impact on mental performance, including decision making! After the match, referees and touch judges should stay for the match supper (if invited!), but should bring suitable refuellers with them to the match, or stop off and refuel on the way home – unless home is just a short journey away and a meal will be waiting for them.

TOURNAMENTS

For players involved in tournaments such as sevens, where several short games are to be played in one day, the priority is to keep restocking energy stores and replacing fluid losses throughout the tournament – or rather, until they are no longer competing. When there are only 30min between games, all a player can do is to use a sports drink, either commercial or home-made, but one they are used to drinking. Water should not be the first choice of fluid as it does not contain any carbohydrate to replace energy losses, nor does it rehydrate as effectively as a sports drink.

Sevens tournaments tend to be played in the summer months when sweat rates will be higher. Although matches do not last long, work rates will be high and sweat rates will therefore also be high. Using a sports drink will speed up hydration and help to prevent cramping in those prone to this problem. For convenience, a ready-made commercial sports drink is probably easier than relying on home-made drinks or gels.

If there are one to two hours between matches most players should feel comfortable having a sandwich. Sandwiches made with white, brown or wholemeal bread are best as they are digested and absorbed more quickly than granary bread. Thin fillings of chicken, ham or tuna are suitable. For those preferring something sweet, honey, jam or banana fillings are also appropriate. With up to an hour before kick-off, cereal bars and bananas can be used to top up energy levels, and jelly beans and jelly babies should be tolerated right up to the kick-off. However, it is important not to overdo the amount consumed. (Remember how many minutes are played in a sevens match.)

It is worth considering taking supplies to tournaments rather than relying on what might be available at the ground. Event catering is usually aimed at the crowd, rather than the players, and eating chips, pies and burgers during the day will certainly not win sevens tournaments.

AWAY MATCHES

League away matches can involve anything from a local derby to an overnight stay in a hotel at the other end of the country. The dietary preparation for a local away game will be more or less the same as for a home game. Players should follow their same meal pattern for the time of the kick-off as for a home match, though perhaps a little more organization will be needed to ensure that suitable fluids and even some simple carbohydrate boosters are available on the team coach, or that individual players have such items with them if they are travelling by car to the away ground. The usual sports drink, cereal bars and some jelly babies or jelly beans should suffice.

Team management should make provision for fluids and food in the changing room in the same way that they do for a home match. What happens next will depend on what, if anything, the home team provides after the

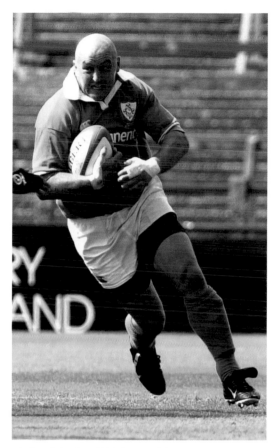

Ireland hooker Keith Wood in action against Wales during the international friendly match at Lansdowne Road, Dublin, in 2003 after returning from injury. (© PA Photos)

Suitable Snacks for Travelling

- Fresh fruit, especially bananas
- Dried fruit
- Cereal and muesli bars and flapjacks
- Sandwiches, rolls or bagels with low fat fillings*
- Fruit buns and scones
- Pretzels, Snack-a-Jacks and Twiglets
- Low fat milk shakes
- Water, fruit juice and sports drinks

* The pre-season questionnaire should help in ensuring a range of fillings to meet everybody's preferences.

match. This could be anything from a sit-down meal to nothing. It is therefore advisable that the team management finds out before the match so that alternative arrangements can be made if necessary.

For longer journeys to away games, more substantial snacks should be provided by the club or the players themselves. High fat foods such as chocolate, crisps, sausage rolls and pies should be avoided. The aim of these snacks is to top up energy levels after the last meal with carbohydrate-rich items, but to minimize fat intake. Players should enjoy the foods provided and feel comfortable after eating them. Sitting on a coach for a long time does not demand a lot of energy, and care should be taken that players do not consume more than they need through boredom eating.

An Overnight Stay: Catering Guidelines

When away matches involve staying the night before at a hotel, it is advisable to contact the hotel in advance to discuss the teams' catering requirements. Hotels may welcome some guidelines about catering for a team of rugby players, and even some suggested menus. Providing general information, together with practical advice on how to adapt meals to meet the specific needs of the players, can help staff provide an enjoyable and interesting menu.

The emphasis of the diet as a whole should be on a moderate to high carbohydrate, a moderate protein, and a low fat content, with neither an excessive nor a low salt content. This is different from the advice about healthy eating. Carbohydrates should be a mixture of starch and sugar, and without any undue emphasis on high fibre foods. Thus there is no need for wholemeal pasta and brown rice to be used, as the overall intake of carbohydrate will be sufficient to provide enough fibre without the use of high fibre foods. In fact high fibre foods can make the diet too bulky, with the result that insufficient energy is consumed. Constipation is one of the main reasons for recommending an increase in fibre intake, but this is a condition that doesn't usually worry rugby players.

As many players do have genuinely high energy (calorie) requirements, it is important that they have access to enough food: a flexible approach to portion control is therefore necessary. Offering meals in a buffet style allows players not only to choose what they want to eat, but how much, as well.

Similarly all players have high fluid requirements, and there should be plenty of fluids available at all times, ideally by providing jugs of water on the dining tables. Plenty of bottled water should also be provided in the bedrooms, either by the hotel or the team management or the players themselves.

The fat content of meals can be kept low in a variety of ways, for instance by using semi-skimmed milk for drinks and cereals, and skimmed milk in cooking if appropriate. The choice of spreads for bread, rolls and toast should include polyunsaturated margarine, butter and a low fat spread. Fats such as butter should not be added to served vegetables, and ideally players should not even be given the option to have cream on desserts and in coffee. Low fat yogurt or fromage frais can be used in desserts instead.

Vegetable oils that are high in unsaturated fats – for example sunflower, safflower, walnut, soya, maize (corn) and olive oil – are the best ones to use in cooking, but even so usage should be kept to as little as possible. Frying should be kept to an absolute minimum and ideally not used at all; for instance, meat should be sealed without the addition of fat. Cream should not be used in cooking; 'creamy' sauces can be made by using skimmed milk, yogurt, vegetables and the minimum of fat.

Grilling, baking, poaching, baking, steaming and stir-frying with the minimum of oil are the best cooking methods to employ as they do not require fat to be added during the cooking.

Where cheese is used in cooking, the use of strongly flavoured cheeses can reduce the total amount that is needed to give the right flavour. Curd cheese and low fat soft cheese are both versatile, low fat cheeses that can be useful in cooking.

Fish (both white and oily), chicken and turkey are all good choices because of their low fat contents. The skin of poultry and visible fat on red meat should be discarded to reduce the fat content even further, and the fat content of gravies kept as low as possible.

Dressings for salads should be low fat/oil free, based on yogurt, herbs, spices, tomato juice, vinegar or lemon juice rather than mayonnaise. If it is feasible players should be able to add their own dressings.

Choices of dessert should concentrate on fruit- and milk-based ones such as crumbles, summer pudding and rice pudding.

The carbohydrate content of the meal can be improved by offering plenty of bread (French, granary, white or wholemeal) and rolls at all the meals. Potatoes should be kept fairly plain by putting boiled, mashed and jacket potatoes on the menu rather than roast, chips or potato 'dishes'.

As an alternative to potatoes, rice and pasta dishes can be included on the menu as long as the accompaniments are not high in fat. Salads can be based around pasta, rice, beans.

A good assortment of cereals at breakfast time should keep most players happy.

Generally plenty of fresh fruit (especially bananas), fruit juice and yogurt should be available at all meals, not just breakfast.

Overall the emphasis at all the meals should be on simple food and plenty of it, rather than rich foods, fried foods, pastry and rich desserts such as gateaux, tortes and mousses.

As players come in a variety of sizes, those catering for them should not be surprised by the variation in appetite, too. Some players may even require second helpings.

Finally there should be a good choice of fluids at every meal, including at least plentiful amounts of water and squash on the tables.

TRAVELLING ABROAD

Although international teams will travel abroad for cup matches and tournaments, many other teams also compete abroad, including touring school teams. Most international teams will stay in smart hotels enjoying appropriate meals that are planned well in advance by the team management and hotel, and which bear remarkable resemblance to meals consumed at home.

Hotel Menu Suggestions

Evening meal

Starters
- Thick vegetable soup (leek and potato, carrot and coriander, lentil, minestrone)
- Low fat fish pâté (using fromage frais or yogurt) served with toast
- Fruit juice
- Plus plenty of bread rolls

Main course
- Roast lamb served with mint sauce and redcurrant jelly and whole jacket potatoes (that is, not cut in half and no added butter or margarine) with lightly boiled or steamed vegetables (again, no added butter or roasted vegetables)
- Poached chicken with a low fat sauce (not a creamy or oily sauce) served with plain boiled potatoes or rice and vegetables as above
- Pasta with a simple light tomato and vegetable sauce (no cream or oil)

Dessert
Fresh fruit salad
Fruit crumble with custard
Rice pudding served with a fruit compote

Breakfast
This meal should not present any problems, and players might be offered the following choices:
- Cereals – any varieties, including porridge
- Semi-skimmed and skimmed milk
- Fruit – bananas and dried fruit
- Toast, rolls, muffins (English not American)
- Honey, jam and marmalade
- Low fat spread, margarine and butter
- Baked beans, grilled tomatoes, poached mushrooms, eggs (scrambled, boiled or poached) and lean, grilled bacon
- Plain boiled pasta (or alternatively spaghetti in tomato sauce)
- Selection of fruit juices, tea, coffee and water

School rugby trips abroad will be a completely different matter. Particular aspects that need to be addressed include the

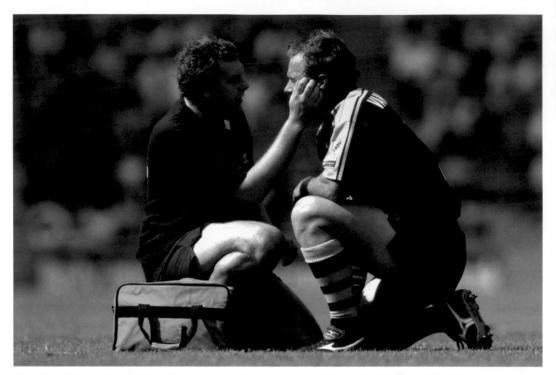

London Wasps' Mark Van Gisbergen receives treatment from physio Roger Knibbs. (© PA Photos)

journey, possible jet lag, unfamiliar food, emergency rations, and food and water safety.

Air Travel

The atmosphere in aircraft cabins is very dry because of the low humidity; in particular this means that players will have to pay special attention to their fluid intake during the flight. Ideal drinks include still bottled water rather than sparkling water (which can lead to internal discomfort), juices and soft drinks. Carbonated drinks such as colas and lemonade should be avoided for the same reason. Alcohol should be avoided too, as it will only exacerbate dehydration, as may drinking more caffeine-containing drinks than normal. Depending on the current airline rules regarding what can and cannot be taken on board, carrying at least a litre of water in hand luggage can help a player maintain their fluid intake between the plane landing and arriving at the final destination.

Any special meals should be ordered in advance, and all players should consider taking extra food in their hand luggage, because meal portions, particularly in economy class, are small for most people and will certainly not be enough for young, growing rugby players – or even adult players, for that matter. Cereal bars and energy bars are probably the most practical to take, together with fresh and dried fruit. Some countries do not allow fruit and other foods to be imported, and uneaten items will have to be binned before going through customs.

If it is going to be night-time at the final destination, players should try to get some sleep during the flight. However, if the plane is due to land during the day, it is not advisable to sleep on the plane because this would probably make it harder to get to sleep later. Young players will probably find it easy to keep awake as they will be more excited at the prospect of what is ahead, and will enjoy the in-flight entertainment more than the adults in charge. Arriving at night-time, players should get to bed as quickly as possible. If it is daytime, players should have no more than an hour's sleep, have a cool shower, and then soldier on until it is 'bedtime' in their new environment.

Jet Lag

The body clock encourages sleep at night and activity during the day. At home the body clock remains stable and is not normally affected by short-term changes in lifestyle or the environment. Flying across several time zones, however, does affect the body clock, resulting in the well-known symptoms of jet lag. These include feeling tired during the day, but being unable to sleep at night, and having difficulty in concentrating or getting motivated. Mental and physical performances are both affected negatively by jet lag. Symptoms of jet lag include headache, loss of appetite, changes in bowel movements and general irritability, and generally symptoms get worse as more time zones are crossed.

The extent to which individuals are affected by jet lag does vary, but young players will tend to be more adaptable than older members of the travelling contingent. Larks or those who enjoy getting up in the morning, rather than owls or those who prefer staying up late, will adjust more easily to an eastward shift, and vice versa. Players who normally have no problems getting to sleep and who are not affected by strange beds, sharing a room, other people snoring, or noise outside the bedroom, will also be less affected. Physically fit people tend to have fewer jet-lag problems than unfit people.

Eating Abroad

Travelling abroad to most countries will present with few, if any risks of gastro-intestinal upsets. Even so, good personal hygiene and food safety awareness are essential if infection and illnesses are to be avoided. Bottled water must be used if the local water is not safe – and even if the tap water *is* safe, some people find that the change from water at home can cause a tummy upset. Ice should be avoided in drinks; teeth should be cleaned with

---

Adjusting to Local Time

- On boarding the plane, change your watch time to that at the final destination.
- Adjust immediately to the meal, bedtime and waking times at the destination.
- Avoid thinking about what would be happening back home.
- Big, heavy meals should be avoided late at night as they may make sleep even more difficult.
- Keep the intake of drinks containing caffeine to the usual amount; certainly do not increase intake.
- Avoid alcohol. Initially it may encourage sleep, but its diuretic properties may require a visit to the lavatory to pass urine and subsequent difficulty getting back to sleep.

---

bottled water, not tap water; mouths must be kept closed in the shower or swimming pool; salad vegetables should be avoided unless they have definitely been washed in bottled or boiled water; and only peeled, but not bruised or damaged fruit, should be eaten. Any meals eaten away from the hotel should only be in well-known establishments, ideally recommended by the hotel manager or people who know the area well. Food should not be bought from markets or street sellers.

Food must be either piping hot or have come straight from a fridge. Foods to be wary of include pre-prepared salads, soft cooked eggs, all fish but especially shellfish, rare meat, hamburgers, stuffed meats, unpasteurized milk, cream, yogurt and ice cream.

Attention to personal hygiene is vital. Hands must be washed before eating or touching food, after nose-blowing, or after a visit to the lavatory. Crockery and utensils must not be shared, and sharing bottles of water or drinks bottles must be avoided at all costs as infections can be easily transmitted this way. Players unlucky enough to succumb to a bout of vomiting and/or diarrhoea must drink plenty of fluids to minimize dehydration. Oral rehydration drinks (for example, Dioralyte or Rapolyte) – made up, of course, with safe water – should be used to replace electrolytes as well as fluid.

Emergency Rations

Suitable food items brought from home can be used to top up food intakes, particularly for those players who struggle with foreign food. Some countries do prohibit the importing of certain foods, such as fruit, vegetables and meats. It is therefore a very worthwhile exercise to find out what is allowed into the particular country that is being visited. Information should be available from the relevant tourist office or embassy. Certainly efforts should be made to find out what sports drinks are available, and if necessary to take out supplies of the team's usual brand.

CHAPTER 5
Gaining Muscle

A sound strength-training programme alone does not increase muscle mass: just as important are an appropriate dietary strategy, sufficient rest and recovery time between training sessions, and adequate sleep. Unfortunately the desire to improve strength quickly leads some players to follow fad diets and to take cocktails of supplements in an attempt to gain muscle rapidly. Outcomes should be measured not only by an increase in bodyweight and positive measurable results from the training programme, but by careful body fat measurements as well. Total bodyweight is not as important as the increase in lean body mass (the mass of body tissue which does not contain fat).

The diet must provide an adequate energy intake, which will probably mean an overall increase in energy (food) intake to cover the cost of building new tissue as well as the cost of the training programme. Inadequate amounts of energy will impair the rate of increase in lean body mass.

Muscle gain is a gradual process, which takes time and patience. For some players, gaining muscle will seem like an impossible task. Everyone has a genetic potential to gain weight as muscle, and if parents are on the slight side, then their offspring will almost certainly be slight too, and gaining muscle could be a very uphill struggle. All players can increase their muscle mass, just for some it is harder, takes longer, and the results are not as great as for those with a genetic predisposition to be muscular. Fortunately rugby does provide opportunities for a variety of different shapes and sizes to take part. However, a scrum half is never going to make it as a prop, and vice versa!

Rate of Gain

It is important to set realistic targets and to monitor progress by keeping a record of bodyweight and body fat composition. Players who are not able to have skinfold measurements monitored can keep a very rough check by just pinching at appropriate places and by keeping a check on waist measurements (*see* Chapter 6). Rate of muscle gain will be faster at the start of the programme, and then there will probably be a more gradual increase over time. Gains do not necessarily happen at a steady rate after the initial increase, and there may even be periods of no gain, even though the training programme and diet remain the same. Players should expect average gains of 0.5–1kg a month once the initial gain has been achieved.

Use the Off-Season

The ideal time to work at gaining muscle is during the off-season or pre-season. For the élite player the off-season is usually about six weeks, and individual players may well be set conditioning programmes to be undertaken during this time. Non-élite players have a longer off-season, and will usually be left to their own devices to maintain some level of conditioning or to at least minimize the loss of conditioning.

For players with a tendency to gain body fat and lose muscle, a balance must be found between enjoying a few weeks of relaxation and being totally inactive, drinking excessive amounts of alcohol and 'enjoying' a poor diet. Gaining body fat in the off-season will make pre-season training much harder and gains that much slower.

THE SCIENCE BEHIND MUSCLE GAIN

To get an increase in muscle a player must be in positive muscle protein balance: in other words, protein synthesis must be greater than protein breakdown. At rest and in the fasted state, protein breakdown is greater than protein synthesis. After exercise in the fasted state, the rate of protein synthesis and breakdown are both increased, but compared to when the player is in a rested state, the net (negative) balance is reduced. This is because the increase in protein synthesis is greater than the increase in protein breakdown. By consuming carbohydrate and amino acids before or immediately after finishing a training session, this situation can be turned around so there is an overall greater increase in protein synthesis and even less protein breakdown, resulting in a net positive protein balance and a gain in muscle.

A number of studies have been undertaken examining the effects of using branch-chain amino acids with or without carbohydrate; a mixture of whey protein, amino acids and carbohydrate; and whey and carbohydrate or casein and carbohydrate before or after resistance training. All these studies have produced positive results. Six grams of protein (a very small amount) consumed immediately after resistance training appears to be enough to produce results.

At the moment it is not clear if carbohydrate alone during recovery from resistance training has the same effect as protein alone, or a combination of protein and carbohydrate. Further investigation is needed to establish if protein and/or protein plus carbohydrate ingested after intense, intermittent exercise helps recovery in terms of muscle protein synthesis, muscle glycogen storage and reduction in muscle damage and soreness during a heavy training programme. Based on the latest research the following recommendations can be made, promoting training adaptations through nutritional interventions (*see* References Chapter 5, 1):

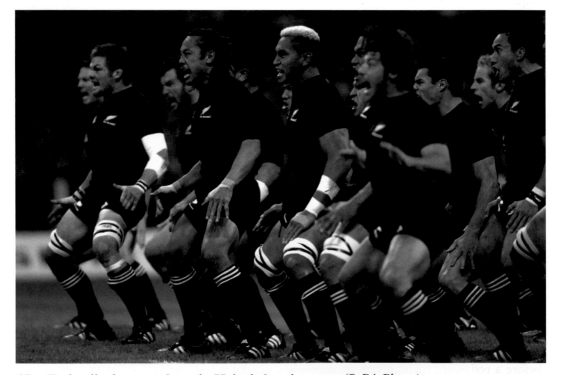

New Zealand's players perform the Haka before the game. (© PA Photos)

- Daily carbohydrate intake during intense training should approach 7g per kg bodyweight per day.
- Nutrient timing before, during and after training can affect many of the adaptive responses to training.
- It is important to provide energy in the form of carbohydrate and/or protein before and within an hour after training.

Certainly there is no new evidence to suggest that high protein intakes are necessary, and the current general recommendations for protein intake still stand (*see* Chapter 2). Indeed, a high protein diet (3.6g or more of protein per kg bodyweight) may actually inhibit the response of muscle protein synthesis to exercise, and is therefore not to be recommended. It is worth remembering that following protein breakdown, nitrogen must be removed from the body by the excretion of urine via the kidneys. Greater protein intakes will require a larger production of urine, which in turn will mean that fluid requirements will increase. Failure to meet this increase will lead to an increased risk of dehydration, which will have a negative effect on performance in training.

Timing appears to be the key to muscle gain, rather than taking in large amounts of protein as food or supplements. In theory, players needing to increase their muscle mass should try to consume 0.5g essential amino acids per kg bodyweight, either immediately before or immediately after their resistance training sessions. However, though most studies have used amino acid mixtures, this does not mean that players should use them. Good quality protein-rich food such as low fat milks, fish, chicken, lean meat and eggs will be just as effective at promoting muscle growth following resistance training.

Of course, using these foods rather than amino acid or protein supplements will also supply other essential nutrients, such as vitamins and minerals, which are needed in the overall daily diet. Players aiming to increase their muscle mass should consider having a small amount of protein (10–20g) shortly before a resistance training session, followed by a similar amount of protein together with carbohydrate immediately after the session. The amount of carbohydrate required will be determined by the player's individual requirement to refuel after training (1.0–1.2g per kg bodyweight).

Suitable Post-Resistance Training Refuellers

The following are examples of suitable immediate post-resistance training refuellers, with approximate amounts of protein and carbohydrate:

80kg player
200g pot fruit yogurt
2 cereal bars
¼ltr sports drink
14g protein and 80g carbohydrate

1 bagel with ½ can (50g) tuna in brine
600ml sports drink
18g protein and 88g carbohydrate

100kg player
1 chicken sandwich made with thick-sliced bread
½ltr sports drink
18g protein and 107g carbohydrate

½ltr milkshake (e.g. Frijj, Nesquik, Yazhoo, Yop or For Goodness Shakes)
6 Jaffa cakes
17g protein and 107g carbohydrate

INCREASING ENERGY INTAKE

To gain muscle, players will need to increase their daily energy or calorie intake by 500–1,000kcals a day. This is on top of the energy intake that maintains a stable bodyweight. The extra energy must be sufficient to cover both the cost of building new muscle and the extra cost of the resistance training programme. The additional food intake should supply carbohydrate to fuel the training sessions, and adequate protein, vitamins and minerals for the development and support of new muscle tissue. Increasing the energy intake is not an excuse for eating or drinking anything that appeals and has a high calorie content. Any ideas of obtaining the extra calories from high fat foods and/or alcohol will unfortunately be very counter-productive.

Food intake should be spread out throughout the day by having frequent meals, mini-meals and refuellers with gaps of no more than three hours between each eating occasion. Eating frequently must become a priority even on the busiest of days. This will require organization and dedication, but it will make it easier to cope with the increased food intake more easily and will reduce any risk of gastro-intestinal discomfort. Gains will

not be achieved by just eating more in an existing pattern of two or three meals a day, and nor will eating in a haphazard way (relying on whatever is available at work, college or school, at the club or gym) lead to the increase in quantity of food that is required, either. Keeping emergency rations in the car, at work or in college or school lockers ensures that suitable refuellers are always available.

Meals should never be skipped, particularly breakfast. Plenty of sleep and rest are important, but breakfast is an absolutely

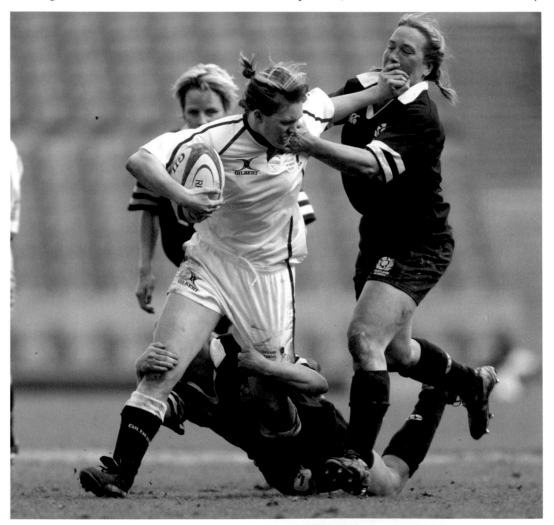

England's Charlotte Barras and Scotland's Rimma Petlevannaya at the Women's RBS Six Nations Championship in 2005. (© PA Photos)

essential meal for all players and particularly for those working hard to gain muscle. Grabbing an extra half-hour in bed and missing breakfast is not a good idea. Instead attempts should be made to go to bed a little earlier.

Portion sizes will need to be bigger, but not to the point where they cause 'internal distress'. A good general guide for the size of meals is to make the largest meals earlier in the day. Bigger meals should also follow harder training sessions, while 'relatively' smaller meals should follow lighter sessions. However, it is still important to refuel and stock up with protein and carbohydrate after an evening training session, even if it is nearing bedtime. Wise choices here include cereal with low fat milk, baked beans on toast or pitta bread, a banana and hot chocolate made with milk, or a chicken sandwich or two. These provide the right nutrient balance but at the same time should not disrupt sleep patterns.

Drinking high energy drinks such as fruit juices, milkshakes or smoothies rather than tea or coffee can push energy and carbohydrate intake up as well as contributing to vitamin and mineral intakes. In the case of milk-based drinks, protein intake will be increased as well, so they can be used as pre- *and* post-resistance training drinks. However, it is better to drink any high energy drinks between meals rather than with them; they can be quite filling, and if drunk with meals, could lead to less food being eaten, which could in turn result in little or no significant increase in overall energy intake. However, fluids do leave the stomach more quickly than solid food, so most players should find they can eat a meal fairly soon after having a high energy drink.

PROTEIN INTAKE

Protein requirements for the general population are based on a sedentary or inactive lifestyle and are set at 0.75g per kg bodyweight per day. Players may need to increase their protein intake up to 1.7g per kg bodyweight per day, which may seem like an enormous increase and could suggest that

protein powders ought to be the order of the day. In fact anybody (including the general population) who meets their energy requirement by including a variety of nutrient-rich foods in their daily diet will undoubtedly also be meeting their protein requirement with ease.

There is no evidence that intakes in excess of 2–3g per kg bodyweight lead to further muscle gains. Such intakes are not harmful, but they can be expensive, and excessive use may mean that other nutritional goals are not met, including provision of carbohydrate. Intakes of protein over and above requirements will be broken down and used either as a source of energy during exercise or converted into body fat and stored.

It is also important not to choose protein sources that introduce a large amount of fat into the diet, particularly saturated fat. Including high fat foods in the daily diet can lead to overall energy intakes that are greater than those required, and rather than seeing a gain in muscle, a more obvious gain in body fat is more likely.

The following table shows the quantity in weight of various common protein-rich foods that provides 20g of protein. Having worked out the required target daily protein intake (bodyweight in kg × 1.7), it should be possible, using this information, to build up a daily protein intake using a variety of different foods.

Daily protein intake

Food	Weight of food	Portion of food
Beef, lamb, pork	75g	2 medium slices
Chicken or turkey	75g	1 small breast
Fish (cod, haddock)	100g	1 medium fillet
Salmon	100g	1 average steak
Mackerel	100g	1 small fillet
Fish fingers	135g	5 fingers
Tuna in brine	100g	1 small can
Prawns, boiled (no shell)	100g	approx 30 small prawns
Semi/skimmed milk	600ml	1 pint
Skimmed milk powder	40g	4 tablespoons
Soy	700ml	A generous pint

Cheddar cheese, reduced fat	60g	2 matchbox-sized pieces
Low fat fruit yogurt	400g	2 × 200g pots
Eggs		3 × size 2 eggs
Baked beans	400g	1 large can
Lentils, cooked or canned	265g	6½ tablespoons
Chickpeas, cooked or canned	270g	7½ tablespoons
Red kidney beans, cooked/canned	290g	8 tablespoons
Soya mince	100g	3 tablespoons
Quorn mince*	165g	6½ tablespoons
Quorn sausage*		3
Quorn burger*		2
Tofu, steamed	250g	
Complan**	⅓ pint	8.8g
Build-up**	⅓ pint	8.8g

* For other Quorn products, refer to on-pack information

** Made up with 200ml or ⅓ pint semi-skimmed milk according to directions – any variety of either product

Protein-rich foods such as nuts and seeds will not be eaten in large enough amounts to contribute 20g protein. However, they are still useful sources of protein, and it is worth noting how much needs to be eaten to provide 10g protein.

	Weight of food	Portion of food
Brazil nuts	70g	21 nuts
Cashew nuts	50g	50 whole nuts
Plain peanuts	40g	30 whole nuts
Peanut butter	40g	thickly spread on 2 slices bread
Seeds	50g	
Trail mix (average)	50g	
Walnuts	70g	21 halves
Seeds	100g	

Some of the protein requirement will be met by the foods included in the diet mainly for their carbohydrate content such as bread, pasta, rice and breakfast cereals. The amount of protein from carbohydrate-rich foods will account for about 10 to 15 per cent of the protein intake, and this must be included when working out the daily protein intake. For example, a player attempting to gain muscle and who weighs 100kg will need a daily protein intake of up to 1.7g protein per kg bodyweight per day, thus a daily total of 170g protein. Between 17g and 25g of this total will be contributed by the carbohydrate content of the diet, leaving 145g to 153g to be provided by protein-rich food and drinks.

Keeping Hydrated

Dehydration will affect performance in the weights room and be counter-productive to weight gain. Research has shown that properly hydrated, resistance-trained weightlifters could lift more than those who were dehydrated. (*See* References Chapter 5, 2.) Passive dehydration achieved by two hours in a sauna and resulting in a loss of body mass of 1.5 per cent adversely affected a one repetition maximum bench press. It is therefore important that players are well hydrated before undertaking weights sessions if they are to get as much as they can out of these sessions.

Players should consume fluids throughout the day, paying particular attention to their intake two to three hours before, as well as immediately after the session. Consuming a sports drink during and after training will maintain hydration status, but it could help in the prevention of muscle cramps, too.

Dietary Fibre

Although the general population is being encouraged to include more dietary fibre (non-starch polysaccharides) for a variety of health reasons, such advice is not appropriate for people who have high carbohydrate requirements. Including large quantities of fibre-rich foods can limit overall food intake because of their bulky and filling nature. Dietary fibre requirements will be met easily just by the sheer volume of carbohydrate-rich foods consumed, regardless of their dietary fibre contents. In fact, a high dietary fibre intake restricting overall food intake would certainly be counter-productive when the goal is to gain muscle.

Practical Ways to Increase Protein and Carbohydrate Intakes

- Make certain that carbohydrate and protein are consumed as soon as possible after all weights sessions: for example milk, milk shakes, sandwich (e.g. chicken, ham, tuna, egg) or an appropriate protein shake and a banana if this is more convenient – or, of course, a properly balanced meal.
- Ensure good quality protein with all meals – lean meat, chicken, fish, milk and eggs. Vegetarians will get their protein from milk, eggs, beans, lentils, quorn, tofu, nuts and seeds.
- When possible, include two protein fillings in sandwiches, rolls and so on: for example ham and cheese, egg and lean bacon, tuna and egg, hummus and chicken, tuna and sweetcorn, low fat soft cheese and chicken.
- Drink more milk.
- Add dried skimmed milk powder to any suitable drinks or meals.
- Make up milk shakes using semi-skimmed milk, extra dried skimmed milk and a milk shake powder to add flavouring. Alternatively use a commercially available milkshake product: Frijj, Nesquik, Yazoo, Yop, Nesquik or For Goodness Shakes
- Use Build-Up or Complan (complete meals) as mini-meals between main meals, making them up according to the manufacturer's directions.
- Snack on dried fruit, milk-based drinks, yogurt, nuts and seeds as well as sandwiches with protein fillings and toast with peanut butter and jam.
- Use concentrated sources of carbohydrate whenever possible such as jam, honey or marmalade on toast; golden syrup or brown sugar with porridge (made with milk rather than water); sugar, dried fruit or bananas with breakfast cereals; additional seeds and nuts with breakfast cereals too.
- To avoid excessive consumption of foods high in dietary fibre, use white bread rather than wholemeal, cornflakes rather than bran flakes.
- Avoid excessive consumption of low energy/ calorie-dense food and drinks.

PRACTICAL TIPS TO GAIN MUSCLE

If weight gain is very slow or non-existent then it is worth keeping some form of food diary. Too often players believe they are eating well, but a carefully kept food diary shows otherwise. Often those who seem unable to gain weight are also the very people who are not enormously interested in food. They may miss meals without being aware of it. When asked the question, 'If you are busy doing something and it is lunchtime, would you break off to have a meal, or continue finishing what you are doing and then perhaps miss that meal altogether?' they invariably answer they would carry on doing what they were doing. Keeping an 'honest' food diary can be a revelation to them.

Such players must try to become more organized by planning each day's meals, mini meals, refuellers and fluids in advance. Make sure that store cupboards, fridges and freezers are always well stocked with suitable foods: this means that a nutritionally well-balanced meal can always be put together.

Some time and effort will be needed, but it can help to keep a running shopping list going: thus as stores of items begin to run low, players can add them to the shopping list, thus ensuring that they never run out completely. For the player who is more enthusiastic about cooking, indulging in some batch cooking (making up quantities for more than one meal) and then freezing meal-sized portions can be very time-saving. However, it is important to remember to take the meal out of the freezer and allow it to defrost before reheating it thoroughly.

Getting as much sleep as possible and trying to fit some rest and recovery time into the day will be a lot easier for some players than others. Sitting at work, college or school, watching TV or DVDs, or lying on a bed just listening to music, all count towards rest and recovery time. Getting enough sleep will probably not be a problem for most players, although some will find it difficult to get sufficient sleep on a regular basis.

Some aspects of lifestyle may be difficult to change, such as those players with jobs that demand they work shifts, including night shifts. Many players may find that sharing rooms with other players leads to sleep difficulties, and others find that sleep patterns become disrupted by non-rugby aspects of their lives. For practical ways to help overcome or reduce sleep problems, *see* Chapter 2.

Muscle gain will only happen if a sound training programme is being followed, the diet is providing sufficient energy, and intakes of protein and carbohydrate are correct in terms of quantity and timing, and there is sufficient rest and recovery time for the adaptation to take place. Only if all these aspects of muscle gain are in place should supplements be considered. (For more information about supplement usage in muscle gain, including the use of creatine, *see* Chapter 7.)

Finally, some patience will be needed. Muscles take time to grow.

CHAPTER 6
Losing Body Fat

Rugby is a sport that now demands players to be fitter, faster and stronger. Gone are the days when forwards and backs could be easily distinguished by physique, and a sprinting forward was a rare beast. Bodyweight and body composition are now monitored closely during pre-season training, and indeed throughout the season at the élite end of the game. Even at non-élite clubs, squad members may be weighed at periodic intervals throughout the season, and individual players may weigh more regularly in the privacy of their own homes.

Bodyweight influences the speed, power and endurance of a player, and excess bodyweight as body fat can have a negative impact on performance, causing a reduction in acceleration and an increase in the physical cost of exercise. In other words, a player has to work harder and is therefore more likely to fatigue sooner. Genetics also plays a part in determining how successful a player will be at achieving a particular bodyweight or distribution of body fat.

There are several situations that can lead to an unwanted increase in body fat. During the off-season the physical activity level is likely to drop off considerably with little or no training undertaken, and yet players may not make sufficient adjustments to their diet to take account of their reduced energy requirements. Players may also see the off-season as a time to relax – quite rightly. However, some may relax their diet too much, indulging in excessive amounts of alcohol, fast foods and rich foods so that the pounds or kilograms pile on.

A player who sustains a long-term injury and is forced into a long period of inactivity may not reduce their overall food intake enough to compensate for the reduction in energy requirements. This situation can be exacerbated by the player turning to alcohol and boredom-eating, for solace. Poor knowledge of the effects of a diet containing too much fat and/or too many take-aways may be the excuse for some players. Fat has very little effect on satiety, which can lead players to what is termed 'passive' over-consumption of calories and a positive energy balance.

For young players it may be a change in circumstances that leads to an increase in body fat. Moving away from home and home cooking to college or university life, with few shopping, budgeting and cooking skills to enable them to cope with catering for themselves, can result in too heavy a reliance on take-aways and fast foods.

Players who do gain weight during the off-season should avoid resorting to fashionable, faddy diets, crash dieting, or the use of products promising quick weight losses. They need to appreciate that it takes time to lose body fat, and that fast weight loss will include loss of muscle mass (and strength) as well as some body fat. Ideally players should avoid, or at least minimize increases in body fat and bodyweight during the off-season, and use pre-season training and an energy-controlled diet that will preserve muscle to achieve an acceptable bodyweight and body fat composition over a sensible period of time.

PRACTICAL ADVICE FOR COACHES

Before encouraging a player to embark on a weight or fat loss programme, coaches should give careful consideration as to whether the reduction in weight or fat is really necessary. They should also assess if it is an appropriate time in the year for the player to attempt the loss, and whether they are setting the player a realistic target weight or body fat level.

Finally they should ensure that the player is getting sound dietary advice, and not being left to their own devices. This might lead to them following a diet that could have a negative effect on performance, or worse, a detrimental effect on health.

MEASUREMENT OF BODY COMPOSITION

Measuring bodyweight alone does not differentiate between fat weight and muscle weight. A gain in weight is usually assumed to be a gain in body fat by the general public. However, players including resistance training as a component of their programme would expect to gain muscle – and therefore bodyweight. Bodyweight alone is therefore not a very useful component of fitness assessments, whereas the body mass index (BMI) reflects body fat stores and is calculated by weighing a player in kilograms and measuring their height in metres and applying the simple formula of weight in kilograms divided by height in metres squared. Individuals can then compare their BMI with the BMI classification.

Body Mass Index Classification	
	BMI
Underweight	< 18.5
Normal	18.5–24.9
Overweight	25–29.9
Obese I	30–34.9
Obese II	35–39.9
Obese III	> 40

While the BMI is easy and very quick to use, it does have serious limitations. The major problem with the use of BMI for rugby players (and athletes in general) is that it uses a single value for simple body mass, and no account is taken of whether this weight contains a large amount of muscle or a large amount of fat.

During a programme designed to increase muscle mass and possibly reduce body fat, bodyweight may stay the same or even increase; so although there may be a favourable change in body composition, the scales will not reflect this. A study of US National Football League players found that although the average BMI for the defensive linemen was 34.6, based on an average height of 1.92m and weight of 127kg, their average body fat was only 18.5 per cent, just within healthy limits for the general population. (*See* References Chapter 6, 1.)

Measuring the skin plus the fat lying directly under the skin with skinfold calipers is the simplest and most commonly used method of assessing body fat, and the measurement of subcutaneous fat depots correlates quite well with total body fat. Measurements should be made by someone who is appropriately trained, identifying the correct sites and using calipers up to the standard of the International Biological Programme and certainly not plastic ones. Five sites are normally recommended, namely the biceps, triceps, subscapular, suprailiac and anterior thigh. There is no need to apply complicated equations to work out the total per cent body fat, as players and coaches will want to see the changes at the different sites and the sum of the skinfolds alongside other fitness test results.

A paper published in 2005 provided an insight into the changes in body composition in Australian rugby league players over their season from April to August, following a pre-season start in December. (*See* References Chapter 6, 2.) Reductions in body fat and increases in aerobic and muscular power were seen during the early part of the season when training loads were highest. Reductions in aerobic and muscular power and increases in body fat occurred towards the end of the season when training loads were lowest, and match loads and injury rates were highest.

When assessing body fat by measuring skinfold thickness is not an option, a simple waist measurement can be a pretty good second best. The player needs to be standing up and breathing out gently. The measurement is taken midway between the lowest rib and the iliac crest (top of the hip bone). The advantages of this method are that it uses bony landmarks to determine where the waist is (not always obvious) and does not require very much undressing on the part of the player. No adjustments for height are necessary, either. Fat around the middle is most dangerous in terms of health, and will not be helping performance either in the gym or on the pitch.

Waist Measurement and Risk to Health		
	Increased risk	*High risk*
Men	94–101cm	102cm and above
	(37–39in)	(40in and above)
Women	80–87cm	88cm and above
	(32–32in)	(35in and above)

THE SCIENCE BEHIND BODY FAT LOSS

The key is to maintain a shortfall in daily energy intake over a period of time. This means consuming less energy than the body needs in order to function properly and to meet the extra energy requirements of rugby training and matches, so forcing the body to make up the deficit by using the excessive stores of body fat. If the energy deficit is too small, body fat loss will be slow or even absent altogether. On the other hand, cutting back energy intake too much will make training sessions very hard as fuel will be in short supply. There will also be a loss of muscle as well as of body fat.

Low energy intakes have a negative effect on performance and health, since they will automatically result in a low intake of carbohydrate, which means that muscle glycogen stores will not be replenished fully after training and matches. The immune system will be suppressed, making a player more susceptible to catching a cold or contracting other types of infection. Overall such a low intake will not support training. The only factor in favour of such diets is there is usually very poor adherence!

A daily energy shortfall of 500kcals (2,100kJ) will lead to a weekly loss of 500g, approximately 1lb of body fat. Doubling the energy deficit to 1,000kcals (4,200kJ) will double the fat loss. Daily intake should certainly not fall below 30kcal per kg fat free mass if impairment of metabolic and hormonal function and health are to be avoided. Careful consideration should be given to carbohydrate intake as insufficient intake can have disastrous effects on training. Players who cut back too much will find it hard to finish training sessions. As their very limited stores of muscle glycogen run out (much sooner than their team mates) they will adopt poor techniques in training and also find it much harder to concentrate. Low glycogen stores put a player at increased risk of injury, and the immune system will also be compromised.

Fat seems to be the key energy-providing nutrient that undermines the body's weight regulatory system. There is nowhere to store alcohol, and as it is essentially a toxin it must be oxidized as quickly as possible. While this is happening the rate at which the other fuels are oxidized is suppressed. The body's capacity to store carbohydrate and protein is small, and careful regulation is necessary,

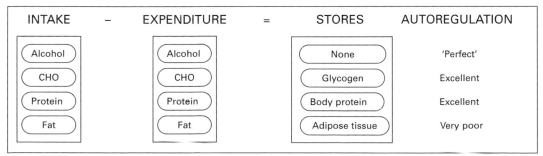

INTAKE	–	EXPENDITURE	=	STORES	AUTOREGULATION
Alcohol		Alcohol		None	'Perfect'
CHO		CHO		Glycogen	Excellent
Protein		Protein		Body protein	Excellent
Fat		Fat		Adipose tissue	Very poor

The regulation of macronutrients in the body.

particularly in the case of carbohydrate. There must always be enough glycogen to maintain blood glucose levels, and yet the liver can only store about 150g glycogen. As a result when more carbohydrate is eaten, more is oxidized, and vice versa.

Fat behaves completely differently, and there is virtually no auto-regulation control of fat balance. When more fat is eaten than is needed, fat oxidation hardly changes, partly because the body's fat stores are virtually unlimited in size. Fat cells can just get bigger and bigger – not unlike blowing up a balloon, except the fat cell doesn't burst! In bygone days, this lack of control of consumed fat was irrelevant, as there was rarely an abundance of food – indeed, in times of famine this would have been a distinct advantage.

Making matters even worse, fat is stored very efficiently with only 4 per cent wastage, compared with 25 per cent when excess intakes of carbohydrate are converted into fat for storage. Aside from the metabolic aspects of dietary fat, people in general will only become fat because of factors that affect appetite leading to overeating in relation to daily requirements. Again, fat seems to take the lead as the poor regulator. Various studies over the years have shown that people gain body fat on high fat diets because they fail to reduce the weight of food they eat. The energy balance mechanisms do not recognize that they are eating fat, and the body does not get the 'stop eating' signs. The result is over-consumption and an excessive intake of calories.

Foods with high water and low fat contents have been shown to help curb appetite compared to those with low water and high fat contents. Fruit and vegetables should therefore win a place in a fat loss diet, and fried and fatty foods ought to get the booby prize. Interestingly our daily diet tends to contain the same volume of food on a daily basis. (*See* References Chapter 6, 3.) Players working at reducing body fat should therefore aim to swop high energy dense foods (fatty foods such as pastries, croissants and crisps) for low energy dense items (fruit, vegetables). In other words, the volume stays the same, but the energy value or total calorie intake goes down.

CAN SUPPLEMENTS HELP WEIGHT LOSS?

There is no shortage of advertisements extolling the virtues of supplements to help weight loss and, more specifically, fat burning. Two such supplements are considered here: L-carnitine and ephedra. Carnitine is involved in the transfer of fatty acids across the mitochondrial membrane inside cells, where they can be oxidized and used as a source of fuel. It is therefore sold on the basis that as L-carnitine increases fat oxidation, it must also be effective in promoting weight loss.

Unfortunately supplementation does not increase muscle stores of carnitine, and it cannot therefore increase the rate of fat oxidation and so will not help weight loss. Moffat and Chelland in their review of carnitine (*see* References Chapter 6, 4) stated:

> In conclusion, the majority of studies reveal that carnitine supplementation does not seem to provide an ergogenic benefit to human performance. The body and diet are sufficient to provide enough carnitine to allow an individual to effectively regulate lipid metabolism both at rest and during various types of exercise.

Ephedra is the herbal equivalent of ephedrine, and is found in Ma Huang. It increases resting energy expenditure, and research data suggests it can help in short-term weight loss. Other ingredients are often found in these supplements, including caffeine and aspirin, green tea and yohimbine. However, before players rush off to their nearest herbalist or health food shop they should be aware of two very serious consequences of using such supplements: first there is substantial evidence of adverse effects when these weight loss cocktails are used, from simple nausea to the worst side effect of all – death. Second, ephedrine and ephedra are both on the prohibited list of the World Anti-Doping Agency (WADA), and the risk of a positive drug test and/or serious health consequences should discourage players from even thinking about using such a supplement, regardless of what level they play at.

HUNGER AND APPETITE

Hunger is the drive to eat, which results from an energy intake that is not enough to maintain energy balance. Real hunger is an unpleasant, even painful sensation directed towards food in general. Appetite, on the other hand, is a pleasant sensation, often the result of seeing, smelling or thinking about particular foods or drinks. For example, having had a particularly enjoyable three-course meal and certainly not needing to eat more, it is appetite that results in an entire box of chocolates being devoured. In contrast it is hunger that will drive people to scrabble in the dust in time of famine. Both represent a desire to consume food or drink but the hungrier one is, the less it matters how appetizing the food may be, and vice versa. Keeping some degree of control over appetite is vital if body fat and/or weight loss is to be achieved. High carbohydrate and high protein foods should be chosen, rather than high fat foods. Fat is less satiating and encourages passive over-consumption so no 'stop eating' signals are sent out.

HOW APPROPRIATE ARE POPULAR DIETS?

Weight gain does not happen overnight, and neither does weight loss. Losing weight, or, more correctly, body fat, has to be a gradual

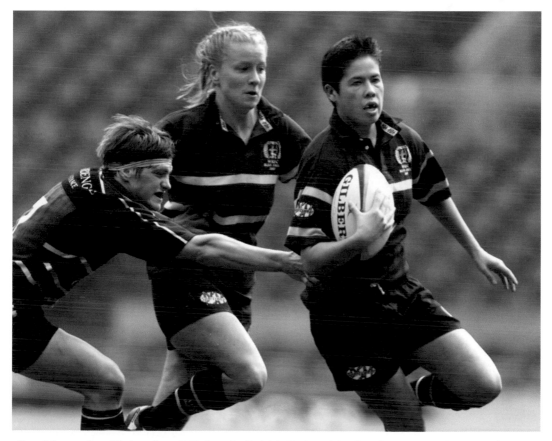

Loughborough v. University of Wales, the British Universities Rugby Union Championship Women's final at Twickenham in 2003. (© PA Photos)

process if it is to be a permanent loss. Quick-fix diets may promise amazing weight loss in a short space of time, but any success will be short-lived. The following diets are popular but are not to be recommended, particularly for rugby players, for reasons that will become clear.

Food Combining Diets

Food combining has been popular for decades. It was developed by an American, Dr William Hay, in the 1900s, not as a weight loss diet or to cure disease, but as a way of helping the body to heal itself. Dr Hay was convinced that many diseases – such as arthritis, indigestion, allergy and intolerance – were caused by the wrong chemical conditions in the body, which in turn were caused by eating too much meat and refined carbohydrate, poor digestion and constipation. He believed that carbohydrate and protein should not be eaten at the same meal because they required different conditions for digestion – although this assumption totally ignores the fact that the digestive system is perfectly capable of digesting foods containing both carbohydrates and proteins at the same time.

Practically, food combining means that bread, pasta, rice, cereals, potatoes and sugars should not be eaten with meat, fish, poultry and cheese. Many people have claimed to lose weight following a food combining diet. However, it must be understood that weight loss will only be due to the limit on food intake imposed by the restrictions of the diet,

and therefore the reduction in overall energy intake. In fact a study published in 2000 found that food combining diets did not promote any greater weight loss than a normal, balanced diet of equal energy content. (*See* References Chapter 6, 5.)

Players should also realize that such a diet will, by its very nature, limit not only energy intake but also carbohydrate intake. This will obviously make both training and matches particularly hard going, as fuel will be in limited supply.

High Protein, Low Carbohydrate Diets (Atkins Diet)

The theory on which most of these diets are based is that they somehow change the way the body deals with food. Supporters of these diets all claim that carbohydrates are the villain and the cause of obesity. They state that dietary carbohydrate causes the body to produce excessive amounts of insulin – the hormone produced by the pancreas, which siphons off glucose from the bloodstream and helps the body to either metabolize it, or store it as glycogen in the liver or muscles. Dr Atkins believed that the hyperinsulinaemia (abnormally high level of insulin in the blood) in turn promoted excess storage of energy as fat. A high protein, low carbohydrate diet is therefore said to lower insulin levels and cause weight loss.

So what is the truth about these diets? In fact, it does not matter how much insulin is in the body, fat storage will not take place unless total energy intake is greater than energy requirements. The significant weight loss that many achieve following high protein, low carbohydrate diets is again due to the consumption of fewer calories than the body needs. It is total energy deficit that has the greatest impact on weight and body fat loss. A diet encouraging a low carbohydrate intake will deprive players of their major source of fuel – and one which the body can only store in limited amounts.

Again, a regular daily intake of carbohydrate is therefore vital if muscle glycogen stores are to be maintained, and hard training sessions fuelled effectively. This is the major

Major Enzymes of Digestion		
Enzyme	*Site of activity*	*Nutrient*
Pytalin	Mouth	Carbohydrate
Pepsin	Stomach	Protein
Trypsin	Small intestine	Protein
Chymotrypsin	Small intestine	Protein
Lipase	Small intestine	Fat
Amylase	Intestinal wall	Carbohydrate
Maltase	Intestinal wall	Carbohydrate
Sucrase	Intestinal wall	Carbohydrate
Lactase	Intestinal wall	Carbohydrate

reason that low carbohydrate diets should not be considered as a way of losing weight – though there are, of course, also the side effects, which include bad breath and constipation. These alone are probably reason enough to put players off trying these diets.

SUCCESSFUL WEIGHT LOSS STRATEGIES

A balanced long-term strategy is necessary, not a drastic quick-fix approach. This can be achieved by targeting the foods that provide plenty of calories but few nutrients, particularly high fat foods and alcohol; and by maintaining an adequate intake of nutrient-dense carbohydrate foods, and lean or low fat sources of protein.

Overall portion sizes may need to be considered, as sheer overeating can often be the cause of an unwanted increase in body fat, even though the actual food choices are perfectly good. A study carried out a few years ago found that putting larger sandwiches in front of young adults caused them to eat more. (See References Chapter 6, 6.) Thus, seventy-five people were given a test sandwich once a week over four weeks. The sandwiches were 6in, 8in, 10in or 12in long, and the subjects could eat as much as they wanted. Most participants finished the 6in sandwiches, but not the others. When the 12in sandwiches were served, men ate 23 per cent more and women 23 per cent more than when served the 8in sandwiches. Hunger and fullness were not different after eating the different size sandwiches.

This study shows that the portion size determines how much people eat. Putting less on the plate can control excess intake – or, better still, use a small plate or bowl: piling up a small plate will obviously mean that fewer calories are consumed than if you were to pile up a larger plate. Snacking out of a bag is probably not a good idea either, as this gives no visual clues as to how much is being eaten. Buffets and barbecues should be avoided as much as possible when trying to lose body fat/bodyweight, as people tend to eat more when presented with a wide variety of foods.

Target high-fat foods such as butter,

General Tips to Reduce Body Fat

- Always eat sitting down, ideally at a table.
- Do not eat whilst watching television or a DVD, or in front of a computer, or watching a film at the cinema, or even just walking down the street. People have no idea either what or how much they are eating when they are doing something else: eating becomes a subconscious habit if they are focused on something else.
- Eat slowly. People tend to eat less if they do not rush their meals – up to 15 per cent less in some cases. Eating quickly does not give the brain a chance to send messages that enough food has been eaten, with the result that the messages to stop eating come through when too much has already been consumed.
- Between mouthfuls put the knife, fork and/or spoon down, as this can help in eating more slowly, and thus prevent overeating.
- Finish chewing and swallowing before putting more food on the fork.
- If eating with other people, talk a lot!
- Some people find writing down everything they eat helps to prevent overeating.
- If the weight loss slows down, do not start missing breakfast as this can lead to mid-morning snacking and a bigger lunch. Also, metabolism slows down overnight, and eating in the morning speeds it back up.
- Remember, weight or body fat loss does not happen at a steady rate week by week.

margarine, cream, full fat milk and high fat cheeses, fat on/in meat, pastry and fried foods. For more information about reducing fat intake, see Chapter 2. Concentrate on carbohydrate and protein, as they are much stronger appetite suppressants. Eating a high carbohydrate/low fat breakfast every day will help to reduce the urge to over-eat during the morning.

Sugar is a form of carbohydrate and can be included in a weight/fat loss diet. A large European study has shown that a low fat/high carbohydrate diet, where the carbohydrate consisted of a mixture of starch and/or sugar, is effective in promoting weight loss. (*See* References Chapter 6, 7.) This study compared subjects who were consuming a diet low in fat and high in carbohydrate (starch *and* sugar) with subjects consuming a diet low in fat and high in starch only. Both groups lost weight, and there was no difference in weight loss between the groups. The authors concluded that it was not necessary to exclude the sugar component of carbohydrate from a weight-reducing diet – and in fact *including* some sugar can improve the palatability of the diet, and of course provide a vital source of energy for rugby players, whether they are attempting to lose body fat or not.

Combine smaller portion sizes with more 'eating' occasions, as going long periods without food invariably leads to a bigger calorie intake than the little-and-often approach would achieve.

Eating Habits and Risk of Obesity	
Change to risk of obesity	
Eating at least one midday snack	−39%
Eating the largest meal in the evening	+6%
Waiting more than three hours for breakfast after waking	+43%
Eating more than a third of meals in restaurants	+69%
Going to bed hungry (three or more hours after last eating)	+101%
Eating breakfast away from home	+137%
Not eating breakfast at all	+450%

Including plenty of fruit and vegetables in the daily diet is not only sound nutritional advice, it can also help in body fat loss. These foods provide bulk but with few calories, so a player will feel full for longer and so delay hunger pangs.

Starting a meal with soup can also help control food intake. Recent research has shown that people who ate a first course of soup before a lunch entrée reduced the total calorie intake of their meal by a fifth, compared with those who ate the entrée

alone. The soup of course has to be low calorie (100–150kcals per serving): having a creamy soup instead would have the opposite effect, boosting calorie intake and leading to weight gain. Similar results have been obtained by blending vegetables into a pasta sauce.

Alcohol intake should also be carefully controlled, as drinks add calories with little or no nutritional value. (*See* Chapter 2 for more about the effects of alcohol on health and rugby performance.)

Sleep

Perhaps Paul Gascoigne was on the right tracks when he took himself off to bed in an attempt to lose weight. According to a study published in the journal *Sleep*, an extra hour of sleep every night may help in weight loss. (*See* References Chapter 6, 8.) People who slept for nine hours or more had, on average, a significantly lower BMI than those who slept for five hours or less. Insufficient sleep increases levels of ghrelin, a hormone responsible for hunger feelings, and decreases the levels of leptin, a protein that helps in regulating appetite and bodyweight. Sleeping for four hours or less also increases the levels of cortisol, helping to trigger carbohydrate cravings.

It is important that by concentrating on body-fat loss players do not lose sight of the principles of the training diet and hydration strategies as discussed in Chapters 2 and 3. A possible solution is to adopt a body-fat loss diet based on the glycaemic index of carbohydrate foods, a plan which the author has used successfully with players who have needed to reduce body fat while maintaining overall performance in training and matches.

A Low Glycaemic Index Diet

A low GI diet involves making changes to the overall diet in terms of *what*, rather than *how much* is eaten, which means there is usually no need for tedious weighing out of food. What will have by far the most impact on reducing body fat will be the *type* of foods consumed, rather than the amount. As fat is

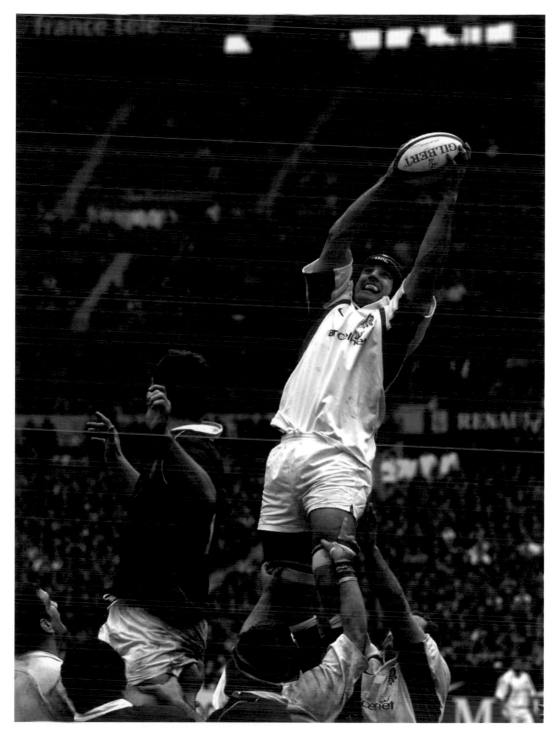

England's Ben Kay takes the ball during the match between France and England at the Stade de France in 2002. (© PA Photos)

the most calorific part of the diet it is important to trim back intake if necessary. The diet plan concentrates on the type of carbohydrate consumed at particular times in the day. The glycaemic index (GI) of a carbohydrate food determines how quickly that food is digested, and how quickly the breakdown product glucose is absorbed into the bloodstream.

When glucose enters the bloodstream it causes a release of insulin. Insulin has two powerful actions: it opens the flood gates so that glucose can move quickly into the cells and be used as a source of energy; and it inhibits the release of fat from fat stores. By having predominantly low GI foods the huge and rapid rise in blood glucose is avoided. As a result there is no large release of insulin, and so the body is forced to burn body fat to meet its energy requirement. Low GI foods help to keep hunger pangs at bay, whereas high GI foods do not. This explains why feelings of hunger bubble up again soon after eating high GI foods.

In the following plan all meals are based

Meal Plan

Suggestions are made for breakfast, lunch and an evening meal each day, as well as some simple snacks. However, these meals can be interchanged or repeated, just as long as no meal occasion is missed out on any day. If a meal does not follow training within 30min to an absolute maximum of 60min, a refuelling snack will be needed; ideally this should contain predominantly carbohydrate with a small amount of protein. This can be achieved simply by having a chicken, tuna or lean ham sandwich using white or wholemeal bread – both high GI foods. Fat content should be kept low, so the addition of mayonnaise or salad cream should be avoided. Buying a sandwich 'to go', players should choose the healthier varieties that are sold in all supermarkets and some garages; these may even be labelled according to their GI value.

DAY ONE

Breakfast
- Porridge made with water or semi-skimmed milk or half milk and half water
- *or* muesli, fruit and fibre, oat and wheat-type cereals
- Glass of unsweetened orange juice
- Granary or multigrain bread or toast with a thin spread of crunchy peanut butter rather than ordinary butter or margarine (it contains more protein than ordinary butter or margarine)
- Tea, coffee or water to drink

Lunch
- Bread (as breakfast)
- Low fat spread, e.g. Flora light, or supermarket equivalent
- Tuna in sunflower or olive oil, drained and mixed with a little vinegar or low fat yogurt, but no salad cream or mayonnaise
- Salad vegetables in the sandwich or as a side salad
- Fresh fruit – any, including bananas
- Fluids of choice – water, low sugar squash, tea, coffee

Evening meal
Chicken stir-fry with noodles
- A little oil or spray-on oil
- Chicken breasts, cut into bite-sized pieces
- Stir-fry vegetables or just suitable vegetables of choice in unlimited amounts
- Sauce, e.g. Blue Dragon
- Quick cook noodles (straight to wok)

Heat the oil, add the chicken and cook until no juices run out when pierced. Add the vegetables and stir-fry for 2–3min. Add the sauce and stir-fry for 1min. Add the noodles and stir-fry for 1min.
- Fluids of choice – water, low sugar squash, tea, coffee
- 200g pot low fat fruit yogurt and a piece of fruit

DAY TWO
Breakfast
As Day One

Lunch
- Bread (as breakfast)
- Omelette made with a little semi-skimmed milk and grated half-fat cheddar cheese; use a little oil for cooking or spray-on oil and ideally a non-stick pan
- Or scrambled eggs with a piece of cheese on the side or grated on top
- Any salad vegetables as a side salad
- Fruit and fluids *as Day One*

Evening meal
Chilli con carne with rice
o A little oil, or spray-on oil
o Onions, chopped
o Very lean mince
o Tomato purée
o Canned tomatoes
o Chilli powder and salt to taste
o Red kidney beans, canned in water, no sugar, washed and drained

Heat the oil, cook the onion until soft, then add the meat. Cook until the meat has browned, add the purée, then the canned tomatoes, and flavour with chilli and salt. Leave to cook gently for about 20min or until the meat is thoroughly cooked. Meanwhile start cooking the rice. Add the beans and allow to heat through while the rice finishes cooking.
Serve with basmati rice.
- Fluids of choice – water, low sugar squash, tea, coffee
- 200g pot low fat fruit yogurt and a piece of fruit

DAY THREE
Breakfast
As Day One

Lunch
- Bread (as breakfast), made into sandwiches with...
  - Low fat soft cheese such as Philadelphia light or supermarket own label
  - Lean ham

- Any salad vegetables as a side salad with the sandwiches
- Fruit and fluids *as Day One*

Evening meal
Chicken special
o Chicken breasts
o Small amount of sunflower oil, or spray-on oil
o Onion, chopped
o Juice of 1 lemon (optional but nice)
o Low fat soft cheese
o Mushrooms, sliced

Slice the chicken into bite-size pieces. Heat the oil and add the chopped onion, cook until soft but not browned. Add the chicken and cook for about 3min, stirring to stop it browning. Add the lemon juice and then the mushrooms. Finally add the cheese and stir until it looks like a sauce. Serve with a vegetable and pasta.
- Fluids of choice – water, low sugar squash, tea, coffee
- 200g pot low fat fruit yogurt and a piece of fruit

DAY FOUR
Breakfast
As Day One

Lunch
- Bread (as breakfast) toasted
- Eggs, scrambled with a little milk. Use whole eggs!
- Baked beans
- Any salad vegetables as a side salad
- Fruit and fluids *as Day One*

Evening meal
- Salmon steak, grilled or chicken breast
- Basmati rice
- Vegetable of choice

Flavour a small pot of natural yogurt with a little tomato purée. Heat very gently and pour over the salmon.
- Fluids of choice – water, low sugar squash, tea, coffee
- 200g pot low fat fruit yogurt and a piece of fruit

DAY FIVE
Breakfast
As Day One

Lunch
- Bread (as breakfast)
- Low fat spread
- 200g can tuna in sunflower or olive oil, drained and mixed with a little vinegar if you like (balsamic or wine vinegar)
- Any salad vegetables in the sandwich or as a side salad
- Fruit *as Day One*
- ½ pint semi-skimmed milk to drink
- Further fluids of choice if needed: water, low sugar squash, tea, coffee

Evening meal
Spaghetti Bolognese
o Small amount of sunflower oil, or spray-on oil
o Onion, chopped
o Very lean mince
o Tomato purée
o Canned tomatoes
o Dried mixed herbs and salt to taste
Cook as for the Chilli con carne, above
- Pasta
- Fluids of choice – water, low sugar squash, tea, coffee
- 200g pot low fat fruit yogurt and a piece of fruit

WEEKEND
The aim is to try to eat in a similar way, though this can be harder as there may be less structure than to the week. The most important thing is to keep to the low GI foods all the time, including at the weekend.

Snacks
- Cereal bars of choice
- Fresh fruit, including bananas
- Dried fruit
- Low fat fruit yogurts
- Milk (semi-skimmed milk)
- Occasional small packet of dry roasted peanuts

The following shopping list is intended to make things even easier for players to follow the diet plan.

Store-cupboard items:
Cereal – porridge, muesli or cereal of choice
Jar crunchy peanut butter
Tuna in sunflower or olive oil
Cereal bars
Quick cook noodles (e.g. Amoy)
Stir-fry sauce sachet (e.g. Blue Dragon)
Sunflower or olive oil
Tea, coffee, low sugar squash
Tomato purée
Canned chopped tomatoes
Canned red kidney beans in water and no added sugar
Basmati rice
Pasta – dry, any variety
Canned baked beans
Mixed herbs
Chilli powder
Cartons unsweetened orange juice
Small packets of dry roasted peanuts
Dried fruit

Freezer:
Frozen vegetables of choice

Non store-cupboard items:
Granary or multigrain bread
Semi-skimmed milk
200g pots low fat fruit yogurts
Natural yogurt (optional – *see* Day Four evening meal)
Chicken breasts
Eggs
Half-fat Cheddar cheese
Very lean mince
Low fat soft cheese, e.g. Philadelphia or supermarket own brand
Lean ham
Salmon steak
Low fat spread, e.g. Flora Light or supermarket own brand

Bananas
Salad vegetables of choice
Fruits of choice
Stir-fry vegetables
Onions
1 lemon (optional – *see* Day Three evening meal)
Mushrooms

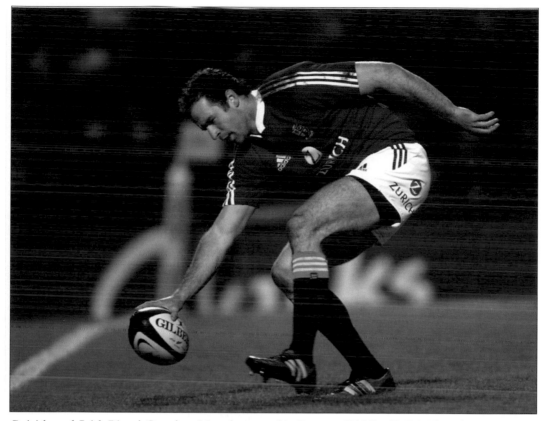

British and Irish Lions' Geordan Murphy scores his first try (2005). (© PA Photos)

around low GI foods – hence particular breads and breakfast cereals, pasta, basmati rice but limited inclusion of potatoes, surprisingly a food that can be moderate or even high GI. Players who miss their potatoes can use sweet potatoes instead as they are low GI foods. Sweet potatoes can also be used instead of pasta, rice or noodles in any of the meals – for a change.

Just before and immediately after any training, players should consume high GI foods and drinks: these will be used as an immediate source of energy in training. Immediately after training they will be used to replace depleted stores of carbohydrate in the muscles. Isotonic sports drinks are a good choice as they not only top up carbohydrate stores rapidly, but of course they also help in the rehydration process. Investing in one of the many books available, or getting information from the internet about the GI value of different foods and brands, will help to add a lot more variety to the diet.

CHAPTER 7

Supplements

Players use supplements for a variety of different reasons. They take them to maintain good health in the hope that they will prevent or reduce time out from training and matches through infections, by boosting the immune system. Some will take supplements to protect their joints, perhaps because they have already sustained a serious knee injury or because osteoarthritis runs in the family.

The decision to take a supplement may be nothing to do with health but all to do with performance, by improving recovery from, and adaptations to, exercise, promoting tissue growth and repair, enhancing energy supplies, delaying fatigue by effects on the central nervous system, or by helping a player to gain muscle or lose body fat, or both. Of course the decision to take a supplement may come about through outside influences such as advice from a coach or member of the training or medical team, from another team member, family friend or well-meaning trainer at the local gym, or just from an advert in a body-building magazine promising instant bulking up. However, all players should be aware that the effectiveness of many supplements has not been proven, and that inaccurate product labelling and poor manufacturing practices could lead to a positive drug test. Some products have less or even none of the active ingredient they purport to contain, others contain substances that are not declared on the label or which are present in much greater amounts than declared. Taking such a product could result in a risk to health and/or a positive drug test.

So why take a supplement? For many élite players it is the pressure to gain every possible advantage over the opposition. For other players it is the belief that diet alone cannot meet all the nutritional requirements. In most cases this is a mistaken belief, and certainly one that can be corrected by sound, practical advice from someone properly qualified to give dietary advice both in relation to health and sporting performance. Players do have increased requirements for energy and nutrients, but this can be met by diet alone as long as the quality, quantity and timing in relation to the type and duration of training are taken into account. However, there are a few supplements that could be beneficial to some players in particular circumstances, and their requirements are as follows:

- They work by influencing the physical, mental or health factors that determine performance.
- They must have no adverse effects on health.
- They must be legal, and not lead to a positive drug test.

SUPPLEMENTS TO KEEP THE BODY HEALTHY

Multivitamins and Minerals

The daily multivitamin or multivitamin and mineral supplement is no substitute for a good diet. For players training regularly and meeting their energy requirements, food intake will be high and deficiencies in these nutrients extremely unlikely. However, this will not be true for the player who misses out whole food groups (such as fruit and vegetables), who exists on a very limited range of foods through lack of time, money or cooking skills, who regularly skips meals, or who relies heavily on take-away meals and convenience foods.

Thus a supplement will never turn a poor diet into a good diet, but it could help to reduce the nutritional gaps while a player works at improving the overall diet.

For a player who does decide to take something, a single multivitamin or multivitamin and mineral supplement is the best choice, rather than a concoction of individual vitamin and mineral supplements. A single supplement will deliver nutrients in the right balance, and provide 100 per cent of the EC adult recommended daily amount (RDA) for each vitamin and mineral. This should be clearly labelled on the packaging.

In the case of some of the minerals, however, the amount will be less than 100 per cent. This is because minerals such as calcium are needed in such large amounts and it is not possible to meet the full RDA in just one tablet. As the supplement is only intended to top up a less than adequate dietary intake, or as an insurance policy, the full RDA would be unnecessary anyway. Players should always use a recognizable brand, and if in doubt as to which supplement they should choose, they should seek advice from a doctor, pharmacist, qualified sports nutrition professional, or even the company manufacturing the supplement.

Having decided to use a supplement, it is important that the player takes it regularly and in the recommended dosage. Forgetful players might like to keep their supplement by their bed or next to the morning breakfast cereal packet as a reminder. Vitamin B2 (riboflavin) is a water-soluble vitamin, which means that any that is surplus to requirements will be excreted in the urine. As this vitamin is a bright yellow colour, this excess will be reflected in the urine colour. This could have implications for the player who is using urine colour to check hydration status. A darkening from the 'normal' bright yellow colour will indicate dehydration – that is, the darker the urine, the more dehydrated the player has become.

Supplements should be looked after in the same way as medicines, and stored safely according to the manufacturer's instructions. It is worrying that multivitamins are often promoted as an aid to optimum nutrition (whatever that actually means). It is certainly not possible to show that supplements promote optimum nutrition if the diet is already adequate. More is definitely not better.

Boosting the Immune System

Regular exercise may have positive effects on the immune system, but there have been concerns that the benefits could be outweighed by the production of free radicals and oxidative stress, which occur during and after intensive exercise. These free radicals seem to be closely involved in tissue and cell damage induced by exercise. The level of free radical production could possibly overwhelm the body's ability to mop up the free radicals before they can do much damage to the muscles. This is most likely to occur during prolonged aerobic exercise, resistance training or when antioxidant defence mechanisms are impaired. However, free radicals also have a good side as they probably help in training adaptations. Antioxidant nutrients neutralize these free radicals, which has led to the theory that post-exercise damage could possibly be reduced by an increase in the intake of these nutrients and a possible speeding up of recovery.

A number of antioxidant supplements have been marketed for this precise purpose. Evidence suggests that they may help in recovery, but it is not conclusive. These supplements usually contain beta-carotene, vitamin C, vitamin E and selenium – all nutrients that can be obtained by including a wide variety of fruit and vegetables in the daily diet, particularly brightly coloured ones. An advantage of using food rather than supplements ensures that not only are these nutrients supplied, but so also is a wide range of phytochemicals. One of the trade-offs of regular training is that the body's own antioxidant defence mechanism becomes more effective. Even hard, intense exercise may not cause any damage in well-trained players, in which case supplementation will be unnecessary once a player is following a regular training schedule.

On the other hand, a player getting by on little training may benefit from an antioxidant supplement as well as increasing fruit and vegetable intake, as could a player at the start of a period of high volume and/or high intensity training. Including lots of different coloured fruits and vegetables (green, red, purple, orange, yellow and white) in the weekly diet is the best way to ensure a wide range of antioxidant nutrients and phytochemicals. Teas (green, rooibos, black), coffee, cocoa, chocolate and red wine all contain antioxidants which will also contribute variable amounts to total intake. Consumption of carbohydrate in drinks before, during and after long, hard training sessions is recommended, as this seems to weaken some of the immunosuppressive effects by inhibiting the release of stress hormones. The amount consumed should ideally deliver 30 to 60g carbohydrate an hour, which can easily be achieved by using a sports drink containing approximately 6 per cent carbohydrate – that is, most isotonic drinks.

Glutamine is a non-essential amino acid found in abundance in the body but particularly in the skeletal muscle and plasma. It is used primarily as a source of fuel by the gastrointestinal tract and the immune system. In particularly stressed conditions following trauma or extensive burns, the requirement for glutamine may not be met by body synthesis alone.

Hard or prolonged exercise can depress the immune system, and some immune cells have been shown to use glutamine at a greater rate as a consequence. As a result, the level of glutamine in the plasma falls, which some have suggested could be restored by glutamine supplementation thereby preventing any impairment to immune function following hard exercise. This theory has not been borne out by research, probably because the fall in glutamine level is small compared to that in trauma or burns patients. After hard exercise the slightly lower level still seems to be sufficient for normal functioning of the immune cells.

Though glutamine supplementation is safe and there appear to be no side effects, it does

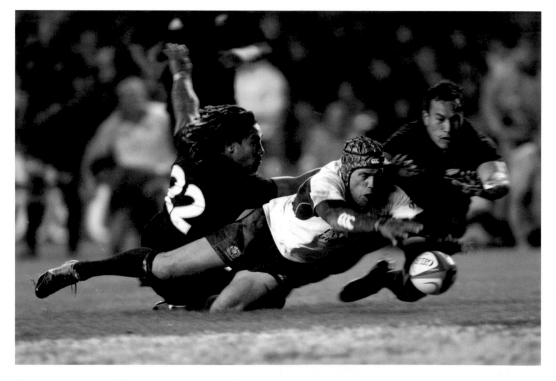

Scotland's Simon Webster scores a try. (© PA Photos)

not seem to be effective in preventing the post-exercise impairment of immune cell function, and players would do better to spend their money on buying food, particularly good quality protein-rich food.

Probiotics

Probiotics are food supplements that contain 'friendly' bacteria such as *Lactobacillus acidophilus* and *Bifidobacteria bifidum*. Regular consumption can modify the population of the gut microflora and influence immune function. Some studies have shown that probiotics may help to improve resistance to intestinal pathogens and limit gut infections. There are no published studies on the effectiveness of probiotic use in athletes. However, players susceptible to gut infections may like to include one of the food products available on the market, which contain these probiotics (for example Actimel and Yakult).

SUPPLEMENTS TO HELP PERFORMANCE

All these supplements are aimed at helping to keep players healthy, but what about supplements that can have an ergogenic or performance-enhancing effect, and which are, of course, totally legal? How can players assess the possible value that a particular product might have on their performance in training and matches? They could try applying the SMART rule.

Applying the **SMART** rule

Safe: Is it safe from a health point of view? Does it definitely not contain a banned substance?

Moonshine: Is the 'science' relating to it rubbish, or accepted fact?

Appropriate: Is it going to be of benefit to a rugby player?

Realistic: Is the dosage and formulation appropriate for a rugby player?

Tested: Are the claims backed up by research, or is the evidence all anecdotal, or relying on celebrity endorsements?

It is vital to check the safety and legality of any supplement, even if the scientific data look promising. The product should not compromise health in any way, or contain toxic or unknown substances or substances that could interfere with other nutrients; and most importantly it should not contain anything that is illegal or banned by the RFU or similar governing body.

Players should not be swayed by endorsements by sporting personalities, but instead should seek advice from a qualified medical practitioner, a registered sports dietitian or a registered sports nutritionist before even buying the product. These people will be able to advise if the product really does what it says, and if it is legal and safe. If, having weighed up the evidence and both parties agree that the player will use a supplement, these professionals will also be able to give advice about how the supplement should actually be used.

Key factors affected by a hard training session that could influence the next training session include fluid and electrolyte losses, depleted stores of carbohydrate in muscles and liver, and a breakdown of muscle protein. Eating appropriate foods will restock glycogen stores and encourage muscle protein synthesis, and drinking a sports drink in sufficient amounts will restore hydration status back to normal.

To Combat Muscle Soreness

Strenuous unaccustomed exercise can cause muscle soreness. This happens soon after exercise finishes, and peaks twenty-four to forty-eight hours later. The severity of the soreness depends on the intensity, duration and type of training undertaken, ranging from mildly annoying to painful, limited movement. Muscle soreness is caused by damage within the muscle fibres, and nutritional advice is to include plenty of foods rich in antioxidants, particularly colourful fruits and vegetables.

Players who habitually have a very low intake of these foods might choose to take a simple multivitamin and mineral supplement or a specific antioxidant supplement – but working at enjoying fruit and vegetables would be even better. The advice to include carbohydrate and protein immediately after resistance training makes sound sense, too.

In Delaying Fatigue

The role of carbohydrate in delaying muscle fatigue is well known, but recent research has also indicated a benefit on central nervous system activities, including cognitive function, mood, motor skill performance, perceived exertion and force sensation. (*See* References Chapter 7, 1.)

The results from a study of twenty active men and women with experience competing in team sports suggested that 6 per cent carbohydrate drinks during intermittent high-intensity exercise, similar to that of team sports, benefited both physical and central nervous system function late in exercise compared with a flavoured placebo. The carbohydrate feedings resulted in faster 20m sprints and a higher-than-average jump height in the final fourth quarter, and also reduced force sensation, enhanced motor skills, and improved mood late in exercise compared to when they drank the flavoured placebo. This is another benefit of using an isotonic sports drink.

Caffeine to Improve Performance

Caffeine intakes are claimed to improve performance, alertness and cognition, and to increase fat oxidation, all of which would certainly benefit a rugby player. Caffeine belongs to a group of chemicals called methylxanthines and is found in tea, coffee, cocoa, colas and other soft drinks, energy drinks and chocolate. It is also found in some over-the-counter medicines including cold and flu remedies, pain relief products, antihistamine tablets and diuretics.

Caffeine is not a nutrient, even though it is regularly found in the diet, but in fact is classed as a pharmacological agent. It is indeed a socially acceptable drug, and the most widely consumed behaviour-influencing substance in the world. It is soluble in water and fat and can therefore appear in all tissues and systems of the body. The liver is mainly responsible for metabolizing caffeine, and the kidneys for excreting it. Peak concentrations of caffeine appear in the blood 30 to 60min after consumption, though the range is wide (15 to 120min). Caffeine has a half-life of between four to six hours. In other words, the highest concentration of caffeine will be in the blood about an hour after consumption, and this level will have fallen by half, four to six hours after consumption.

In the past it was thought that high doses of caffeine were needed to show performance improvements, but a study carried out at the Australian Institute of Sport showed that the amount of caffeine in just two cans of cola was enough to show significant improvements in well trained cyclists in time trial tests. (*See* References Chapter 7, 2.) A review paper published in 2004 looked at thirty-nine caffeine studies, twenty-one involving endurance exercise, twelve involving short-duration, high-intensity exercise and six using a graded exercise test. (*See* References Chapter 7, 3.)

The longer events produced the biggest effects, but improvements were also seen in short-duration, high-intensity exercise. Just small amounts (60mg) of caffeine, equivalent to one cup of coffee, were shown to have effects on decision-making, alertness and reaction time, and 1–3mg caffeine per kg bodyweight were shown to enhance endurance performance. Higher doses in the order of 5mg per kg bodyweight had similar effects to these smaller doses.

A study published in 2005 investigated the effects of caffeine in a performance test simulating physical and skill demands of a rugby union game. (*See* References Chapter 7, 4.) Nine competitive male rugby players ingested either 6mg caffeine per kg bodyweight or a placebo seventy minutes before performing a rugby test. Each test consisted of seven circuits in each of two forty-minute halves with a ten-minute half-time rest. Each circuit included stations for measuring sprint time, power generation in two consecutive drives, and accuracy for passing balls rapidly.

The conclusion from the study was that

caffeine is likely to produce substantial enhancement of several aspects of high-intensity team sport performance, and the final comment of the authors was:

> This effect of caffeine is likely to be important in competitive sports where the ability to perform skills such as passing balls, hitting balls or shooting goals with accuracy late in the event is a key to successful performance.

This would suggest that a caffeine-containing drink at half-time could have a positive effect on performance in the dying minutes of a match, particularly one with plenty of added-on injury time. However, players who take longer for the caffeine to reach peak concentration in the blood should perhaps consider consuming the drink around the warm-up. Overall the literature suggests that small to moderate intakes of caffeine of around 2mg per kg bodyweight, rather than the traditional larger doses of 6mg per kg bodyweight before or during matches, reduce the perception of fatigue and therefore could enhance performance.

Individual responses to caffeine intake, and to the withdrawal of caffeine from the diet, are enormous. Frequent high intakes cause a rapid desensitization in people, which means that more is then needed to get the same result. A sensible approach for players intending to use caffeine in the match situation would be to moderate their caffeine intake on non-match days so that the effect of a larger intake on match days is maximized. There seems no good evidence that complete caffeine withdrawal is necessary, however. (The effect of caffeine on hydration status is covered in Chapter 3.) Players should be aware that although caffeine was removed from the World Anti-Doping Agency (WADA) list of banned substances early in 2004, its use is being monitored in competition, and the situation could change.

Bicarbonate

Lactic acid is produced during high-intensity anaerobic exercise such as sprinting, and the rate of production can overwhelm the body's normal method of getting rid of it. Bicarbonate supplements are widely used by athletes who take part in events that cause fatigue in minutes, such as middle-distance runners. At the moment there does not seem to be any benefit in using bicarbonate supplements in events lasting longer than ten minutes, and in any case the rather nasty side effects that can occur – such as nausea, vomiting, diarrhoea and muscle cramps – would undoubtedly deter most players.

Creatine

Creatine occurs naturally in the body, with the highest concentration in skeletal muscle and about two-thirds of the total in the form of creatine phosphate. At rest the amount of creatine phosphate in resting muscle is three or four times the amount of adenosine triphosphate (ATP), the immediate source of energy for muscle contraction. In normal healthy people, muscle creatine is broken down to creatinine and excreted in urine at the rate of approximately 2g a day. Levels of creatine are constantly replenished by the body making creatine from amino acids in the liver, and also from a diet containing in particular meat, but also fish.

Caffeine Content of a Range of Beverages	
Caffeine content	
Average cup of instant coffee	75mg*
Average mug of instant coffee	100mg*
Average cup of brewed coffee	100mg*
Average cup of tea	50mg*
Regular cola drink	11–70mg per can**
Regular cola drink	16–106mg per 500ml bottle**
Regular energy drink	up to 80mg per can*

* Source: Food Standards Agency advice for pregnant women on caffeine consumption, 10 October 2001.
** Source: MAFF Food Safety Directorate 1998.

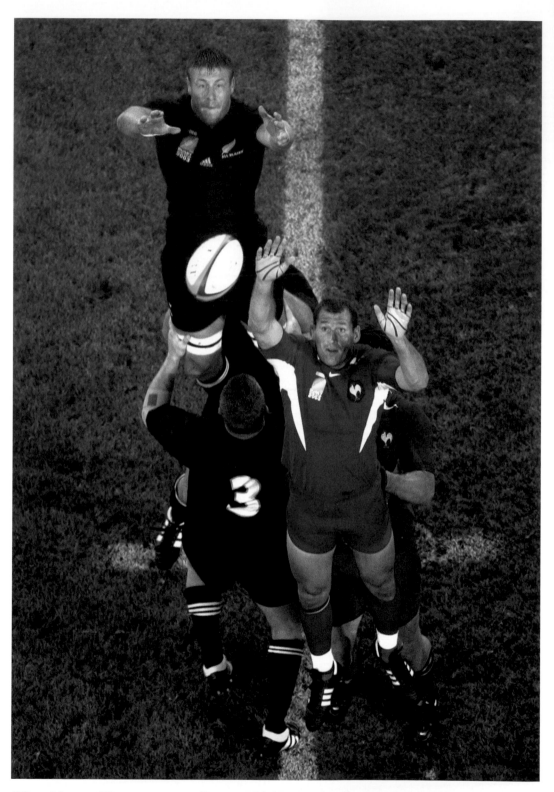

Oliver Magne of France contests a line out with New Zealand's Chris Jack (2003). (© PA Photos)

Creatine phosphate is an important energy source in high-intensity exercise. It is particularly important in recovery between intense bursts of exercise such as sprinting or weight-lifting. Muscle fatigue is associated with a fall in ATP concentration, and if fatigue is to be avoided, the rate of ATP regeneration must match ATP breakdown closely. Rephosphorylation of ADP allows exercise to continue. The ATP content of the muscle rarely falls by more than about 25 to 30 per cent, even when an individual is completely exhausted.

Regeneration of ATP at a rate close to that of ATP hydrolysis or breakdown is essential if muscle function is to be preserved. Using creatine supplements can increase the amount of creatine and creatine phosphate in muscles. The benefits of creatine supplementation should therefore be apparent in training situations such as resistance and interval training, but also in the match situation as well. Several studies have shown that creatine loading enhances exercise performance involving repeated high-intensity bursts of exercise that have only short recovery times of less than 2min between each burst.

Supplements of creatine are available as creatine monohydrate or as salts of creatine, such as creatine citrate or creatine pyruvate. The classical protocol for creatine supplementation is an initial loading phase of 20g a day (in four portions of 5g) for four to seven days. A subsequent dose of 2g a day maintains the high creatine concentration for thirty-five days, whereas if no maintenance dose is taken there is a slow, gradual decline in creatine muscle concentration. There is a slower increase on a dose of 3g a day (without loading), but after twenty-eight days the total creatine concentration is similar to that after rapid loading.

Creatine uptake in the muscles appears to be enhanced if a carbohydrate-rich meal or snack is consumed at the same time. This is particularly relevant for players who have loaded with creatine alone but found no performance benefits. Carbohydrate ingestion is believed to stimulate muscle to take up creatine via an insulin-dependent mechanism. Insulin may stimulate the sodium-potassium

pump activity, and as a result the sodium-dependent muscle creatine transport. Others who have not responded to creatine supplementation have found that by taking creatine with carbohydrate they have also been able to enjoy its benefits.

Although there are little research data about the length of time that supplementation should continue, a sensible approach is probably to have a wash-out period of at least four weeks after supplementing for eight to ten weeks. As vegetarians have no dietary source of creatine they have low creatine concentrations. However, they respond better to supplementation than people who have a higher natural muscle creatine content through eating meat.

Creatine supplementation often causes an initial weight gain of 1 to 3kg within a few days of loading with the supplement. This is almost certainly a result of water retention, rather than an amazingly rapid gain in muscle mass. Further slower increases over about eight weeks will be due to the training that has been achieved as a result of creatine supplementation.

Creatine is not on the WADA list of banned substances, and supplement usage guidelines as already described have been found to be generally safe. The initial concerns that creatine supplementation might have adverse effects on kidney function have been alleviated, as studies have shown no adverse effects after both acute and prolonged creatine intake.

There is no point in using any products that contain anything other than creatine and possibly carbohydrate, as the dosage for creatine use is very specific. It is suggested that players who decide to use creatine evaluate the effects of taking the supplement by keeping a diary to record their bodyweight at the start of the loading phase and the maintenance phase, and any comments about training, and any benefits and/or side effects that could be attributed to creatine.

HMB (Beta-hydroxy-beta-methylbutyrate)

HMB is a naturally occurring by product of one of the essential amino acids, leucine. It has been claimed that supplementation with HMB decreases muscle protein breakdown and therefore contributes to the build-up of muscle, and a consequent increase in muscle strength. A small number of studies have been carried out in the last ten years, but results are at best ambiguous.

A study published in 2003 investigated the effects of HMB supplementation on the aerobic capacity of élite male rugby players. (*See* References Chapter 7, 5.) No difference in aerobic power in the HMB groups compared with the control group at post-trial testing was observed. Parameters of anaerobic capacity improved with training, but there was no difference between the control and HMB groups at the end. However, these results need to be viewed with some caution, as the highly trained and motivated subjects studied were not blinded to the treatments – that is, they knew what they were taking.

There do not appear to be any side effects in short-term usage of up to eight weeks, but there are no present data about usage beyond this period. Overall evidence appears to be weak, and there have been suggestions that more independent studies should be undertaken. HMB is not on the WADA list of banned substances.

NOTES OF CAUTION

Players should avoid taking excessive amounts of many different supplements. Not only is this a very expensive practice, but combining a variety of supplements could change the outcome so that results are not as good as anticipated. Taking cocktails of supplements also raises the issue of safety in terms of overdosing and increasing the risk of contamination.

Inadvertent positive drug tests from the use of supplements can arise in a number of ways. The supplement may contain a banned substance, which is declared on the label, but the player is not aware that it is a banned substance. Or the label may include an ingredient that is not necessarily understood to be a banned substance. For example, a product may include Ma Huang on the label, and not all players will necessarily know that this is actually ephedrine, which is on the banned substances list.

More worryingly, the supplement could contain a banned substance that is not declared on the label. These substances may be added deliberately by the manufacturer, or they may be the result of contamination through poor manufacturing practices. Either way they could lead to a positive drugs test, because the rule of strict liability applies: this means that a player is strictly liable for the substances found in his or her bodily specimen (urine or blood sample), and that an anti-doping rule violation occurs whenever a prohibited substance (or its metabolites or markers) is found in a bodily specimen, whether or not the athlete intentionally or unintentionally used a prohibited substance or was negligent or otherwise at fault. In other words, a player is liable for what is found in his or her body. Blame cannot be passed on to someone else: the buck stops with them.

THE RFU POSITION STATEMENT ON SUPPLEMENTS

Rugby players are strongly advised to be extremely cautious about the use of any supplement because no guarantee can be given by *anybody* that any particular supplement, including vitamins and minerals, ergogenic aids and herbal remedies, is totally free from prohibited substances.

The manufacture of nutritional supplements, ergogenic aids and herbal products may not be subject to the same stringent standards as those applied to the manufacture of pharmaceutical medicines. There is a risk that these products may:

- contain ingredients not listed on the label;
- contain ingredients in different amounts to those listed;
- contain ingredients which are banned substances;
- contain ingredients which are precursors of banned substances.

Consequently the ingestion of these products may increase the risk of a player incurring a positive drugs test, so all players are urged to be extremely careful about which supplements they use.

Remember, a player is solely responsible for any prohibited substance found to be present in their body. It is not necessary that intent or fault on the player's part be shown in order for an anti-doping rule violation to be established, nor is lack of intent or fault a defence to testing positive to a prohibited substance because of a contaminated supplement.

The RFU therefore recommends that:

1. Players should be extremely cautious about the use of any nutritional supplements, ergogenic aids and herbal products.
2. Nutritional supplements, ergogenic aids and herbal products should only be used where the process is controlled and individually monitored by appropriately qualified medical practitioners and nutritionists who are able to screen the supplements used.
3. All nutritional supplements, ergogenic aids and herbal products are taken at the individual player's risk and with their personal responsibility.

USEFUL WEBSITES

www.rfu.com
www.therfl.co.uk
www.uksport.gov.uk
www.didglobal.com (UK Sport drug information database)
www.100percentme.co.uk
www.wad-ama.org

CHAPTER 8

The Young Player

Children and adolescents have dietary requirements that are different from adults, but those involved in rugby at a competitive level will also be different from their non-sporty friends because of the physiological demands of rugby that must be met by their diet: this must support their training and matches as well as their growth and development. However, lifestyle issues can compromise a player's ability to meet these requirements, particularly if their time management skills are poorly developed.

For example, young players may encounter problems over which they have no control, such as inappropriate school meals, in both quantity and quality; excessive travelling time, if they have to go straight from school to training sessions; and financial constraints on the amount of money that can be spent on extra food.

Furthermore, adolescence is a time marked by an increase in independence generally, and this may be reflected in many ways, including a change in eating patterns and food choices which may be to the detriment of both health and rugby performance.

GROWTH IN HEIGHT AND WEIGHT

A person's increase in height happens in four phases. Growth is rapid in the first three years of life, steady in middle childhood, rapid during the adolescent growth spurt, and then slows into early adulthood. During childhood, boys and girls are approximately equal in height, growing at 0.05m a year. Peak height velocity occurs in girls between 11.4 and 12.2 years, and in boys between 13.4 and 14.4 years. Boys have a later growth spurt, but are eventually taller because it is

---

Challenges for Players and Parents

Challenge for the young player
- Understand the link between nutrition and performance
- Juggling training and matches with education, rest and recovery time, family and friends
- Peer pressure from non-sporty friends
- Food availability at all times and places
- Misinformation: who is right and who to believe?

Challenge for the 'older' young player
- Budgeting
- Time management
- Cooking and hygiene skills
- Lack of free time
- Peer group pressure from friends and fellow players
- Alcohol

Challenge for parents and carers
- Understanding the importance of nutrition in relation to rugby
- Fitting meals around the busy timetable of the player and the rest of the family
- Involving the whole family
- Leading by example
- Teaching cooking, budgeting skills etc.
- Being a trainer in life skills

---

more intense. However, there is great individual variation in the timing, rate and intensity of growth in height, as can be seen clearly when looking at secondary school class photographs. Again, peak weight velocity occurs in girls before boys, occurring 0.25 years after peak height velocity in girls and 0.63 years in boys – in other words, boys and girls grow upwards, and then they grow outwards. The weight increase in boys is due to increases in bone and muscle with a levelling off in fat mass. In girls there is an increase in bone, muscle and fat mass.

ENERGY REQUIREMENTS

Children and adolescents have higher energy requirements than adults on a weight basis, because they need to cover the energy cost of growth and development. Absolute energy needs for growth are higher during adolescence than in childhood years.

The extra energy cost of exercise in serious young athletes must be added to the 'Estimated Average Requirements'. The simplest way to calculate the total daily energy requirements is to use the 'Physical Activity Level' (PAL) (see References Chapter 8, 1). An assumption of the energy demands at school/college and during the rest of the day is made, and by using the 'Basal Metabolic Rate' (BMR), estimated average energy requirements can be calculated. A higher PAL value indicates a higher physical activity level.

Estimated Average Requirements (EARs) for Energy (kcal/d)

(See References Chapter 8, 1)

Age in years	Males	Females
7–10	1,970	1,740
11–14	2,220	1,845
15–18	2,755	2,110
19–50	2,550	1,940

EAR for Adolescent Males

The following table shows the 'Estimated Average Requirement' according to bodyweight and physical activity level (kcal/d) for males aged ten to eighteen years. (See References Chapter 8, 1)

Bodyweight (kg)	BMR (kcal)	PAL =1.6	PAL =1.8	PAL =2.0
30	1,188	1,901	2,138	2,376
35	1,276	2,042	2,297	2,552
40	1,365	2,184	2,457	2,730
45	1,453	2,325	2,615	2,906
50	1,542	2,467	2,776	3,084
55	1,630	2,608	2,934	3,260
60	1,718	2,749	3,092	3,436
65	1,807	2,891	3,253	3,614
70	1,897	3,035	3,415	3,794
75	1,986	3,178	3,575	3,972
80	2,074	3,318	3,733	4,148
85	2,163	3,461	3,893	4,326
90	2,251	3,602	4,052	4,502

EAR for Adolescent Females

The following table shows the 'Estimated Average Requirement' according to bodyweight and physical activity level (kcal/d) for females aged ten to eighteen years. (See References Chapter 8, 1)

Bodyweight (kg)	BMR (kcal)	PAL =1.6	PAL =1.8	PAL =2.0
30	1,095	1,752	1,971	2,190
35	1,162	1,859	2,092	2,324
40	1,229	1,966	2,212	2,458
45	1,295	2,072	2,331	2,590
50	1,362	2,179	2,452	2,724
55	1,429	2,286	2,572	2,858
60	1,496	2,394	2,693	2,992
65	1,563	2,500	2,813	3,126
70	1,630	2,608	2,934	3,260
75	1,697	2,715	3,055	3,394

There are few data for children who train regularly in any sport, let alone specifically young rugby players. It is also not relevant to use any data on adult players, as this does not take into account how inefficient children are at using their energy stores. Therefore using these tables would appear to give the best estimate of energy requirements. Practically, monitoring anthropometric measurements such as height, weight (and body fat in older teenagers), fitness testing and overall performance in training and matches will be a reasonable way of assessing if a player is getting sufficient energy.

The quality of the energy (that is, what is actually eaten and drunk) may be a different matter, but certainly poor energy intakes that do not match requirements over a significant period of time can result in growth retardation, delayed puberty, poor bone health and increased incidence of injuries – and of course poor performance in training and matches.

ADEQUATE FUEL

Carbohydrate and fat are both used as fuel

A Day's Food for a Teenage Rugby Player

The following is a typical day's food intake for a nineteen-year-old rugby player.

Breakfast
Large bowl Coco Pops and semi-skimmed milk
1 boiled egg
1 thick slice white bread with low fat spread
Mug tea with milk and sugar
Training: 1ltr sports drink

Lunch
Large French stick with low fat spread and ham
Müllerice
Fruit juice
Training: 1ltr sports drink
Post-training: Banana, milk, Jaffa cakes and
    popcorn

Dinner
2 large chicken breasts
Rice (150g uncooked weight)
Canned chopped tomatoes
Orange squash
Müller corner and Müllerice

Later in evening
Ice lolly
Tea with milk and sugar
3 Mini rolls

Approximate nutritional content
5,000kcals
8g carbohydrate per kg bodyweight
2g protein per kg bodyweight
5ltr fluid

---

sources (substrate), but children use relatively more fat and less carbohydrate during exercise than either adolescents or adults, including during short, intense, more anaerobic-type exercise, as well as prolonged exercise. The results from a study that examined substrate use during exercise in early pubertal, mid-pubertal, late pubertal and young adult males led the investigators to conclude that the development of an adult-like metabolic profile occurs between mid- to late puberty and is complete by the end of puberty. (*See* References Chapter 8, 2.)

To sustain training over a number of months, children still depend on adequate carbohydrate stores to be present. Increasing carbohydrate intake during exercise of high intensity lasting longer than 60min may not only improve performance but also spare the body's stores of fuel for growth and development. (*See* References Chapter 8, 3.) There is certainly no evidence that fat intake should be more than 35 per cent of total energy intake in children or adolescents. Growth and maturation are genetically determined, but a high energy diet will help to maximize normal growth and the effects of the training programme.

PROTEIN REQUIREMENTS

Children and adolescents have slightly higher protein requirements than inactive adults. As the protein requirements of adult players are higher than those of non-active or sedentary adults, it is more than likely that young rugby players have protein requirements that are higher than their less active friends, since protein intake must meet the needs of growth and development, *and* the requirements for rugby. However, as there are no published studies of the protein requirements of young sportspeople in general (and certainly not in rugby), no specific recommendations can be made.

Muscle growth comes from enjoying a high energy diet that provides most of the energy as carbohydrate, good quality protein and other essential nutrients, a well planned training programme, and sufficient rest and recovery time. It also comes with physical

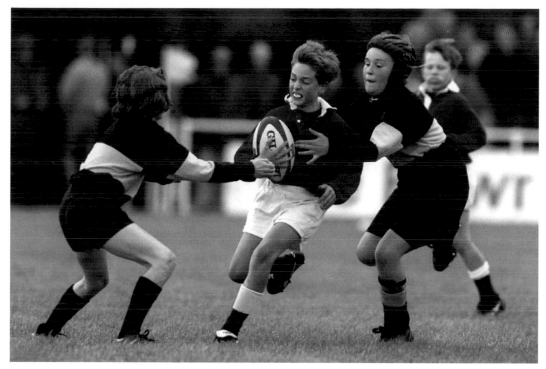

Young boys and girls get their chance to shine on the pitch in a game of mini rugby at Cambridge. (© PA Photos)

maturity, the stage of development when hormones are released in sufficient amounts to stimulate muscle growth. If energy requirements are being met and the diet necessarily contains a good selection of foods, including good sources of protein, protein intake should be enough to meet demands.

Nitrogen balance studies carried out with young footballers (fifteen years of age) indicate a possible daily protein requirement of 1.6g per kg bodyweight. (*See* References Chapter 8, 4.) The practical dietary advice in Chapter 5 concerning muscle gain would certainly be suitable for adolescent players during their growth spurts.

FLUID REPLACEMENT

Serious young players could be at risk of becoming dehydrated during training and matches as they are less efficient at thermoregulation and more susceptible to heat stress than adults. Children are particularly at

risk compared to adults, as they are inefficient at adapting to extremes of environmental temperature, get hotter during exercise, sweat less but have a lower heart output and a greater surface area to body volume ratio. They are also less able to transfer heat from inside the body to the skin than adults, plus they fail to recognize or respond to thirst.

Adolescents adapt somewhere between children and adults. From studies carried out on young footballers it would appear that sixteen- to eighteen-year-olds do not differ significantly from adult male players in terms of the amount they sweat and the amount of sodium they lose during training sessions.

Coaches, teachers and parents can help by making sure that players arrive fully hydrated for training sessions and matches. They should also check that players have their own drinks bottle, containing an appropriate fluid, before the start of all training sessions and matches. Children generally do not instinctively or voluntarily replace fluid losses during exercise, and yet, as already explained, they are at greater risk of dehydration than adults.

Coaches and parents should therefore frequently remind young players to drink. Ideally coaches ought to allow drinks breaks every 15 to 20min – and perhaps more frequently in warmer weather. Younger children should be allowed to drink until they feel their thirst has been quenched, and then encouraged to drink a little more; this is because their thirst mechanism is still not well developed.

Young players who are particularly irritable towards the end of a training session should have their fluid intake monitored to assess how much they are drinking. Flavouring the drink and, where possible, keeping it cool can increase the palatability if this is a major factor in poor fluid intakes. Young players will drink more when it tastes good. In a study of nine- to twelve-year-old untrained boys who exercised intermittently in a hot environment, voluntary consumption increased by 45 per cent when grape flavouring was added to water. Drinking was improved by another 46 per cent when carbohydrate and salt were also added, enough to prevent dehydration. (*See* References Chapter 8, 5.)

Young players should be discouraged from using carbonated drinks before, during and after exercise, as these can cause bloating and possibly lead to insufficient fluid intake. Sports drinks are an excellent source of energy, and fluids during and after exercise, but players should take care to follow the dental advice in Chapter 3 when using them. Drinks bottles should not be shared around among other players, but if they are, they must not let their lips touch any part of the bottle. The drink should be squirted directly into the mouth.

SUPPLEMENTS

Young players may decide to use a supplement for a variety of reasons. They may think it will help to lift their performance when they feel they have reached a plateau. Coaches, parents, team-mates, usage by the first team at their club, advertisements in match programmes or on boards around the ground – all of these could influence young players to try using them. Many are readily available and often advertised as a 'safe and natural' way to enhance performance. In the USA, usage of creatine in adolescent athletes is reported to be 7 to 30 per cent, with even some twelve-year-olds using it. Rather than copying this alarming trend, players, parents and coaches should heed the advice of the American College of Sports Medicine, who advise that creatine should not be used by persons under the age of eighteen years. (*See* References Chapter 8, 6.)

There are several reasons why this advice should be heeded. Children rely more on aerobic rather than anaerobic metabolism, and creatine supplementation – which enhances anaerobic metabolism – will have little, if any, effect. Adolescents seem able to regenerate high energy phosphates during high-intensity exercise, and to improve short-term high-intensity exercise through training, making creatine usage rather unnecessary. In any case, performance during growth is predominantly limited by mechanical factors rather than the relative contribution of the aerobic and anaerobic energy systems. Perhaps most importantly, the long-term safety and efficacy of creatine supplementation has not been established in children and adolescents.

PRACTICAL ADVICE SPECIFIC TO YOUNG PLAYERS

Much of the advice in other chapters will be highly appropriate for the young player, such as the consumption of carbohydrate and protein after any resistance training sessions; the use of sports drinks at appropriate times; and ensuring an adequate intake of iron, calcium and antioxidants. However, there are areas that need to be addressed to take account not only of the added energy and nutrient demands for growth, but also the particular lifestyles that young players enjoy.

Young players need to eat very regularly, and limiting their intake to just three meals a day, even if these are made up of large portions, will not be enough to meet requirements. A daily pattern of between five and indeed up to nine eating occasions (meals, refuellers, light meals, snacks) may be necessary to achieve the required energy and nutrient intakes. Drinks of milk, milk shakes, fruit juices and sports drinks are quick and easy ways of consuming a lot of nutrients and energy in a relatively small volume.

Fluids can help to reduce the potential gastro-intestinal problems that can result from eating a lot of bulky foods, as fluids leave the stomach pretty quickly. However, large volumes of fluid should not be drunk *with* meals as they can limit the amount of food eaten at the meal. Young rugby players certainly do not need to consume high fibre foods. The rather sedentary general population is being encouraged to consume more fibre-rich foods, but such advice is inappropriate for healthy, growing young rugby players. Again, the use of sugar on cereal and in drinks and sports energy bars should not be dismissed for the same reason, as they provide compact sources of much needed carbohydrate.

To help meet energy requirements it is essential to keep a supply of suitable snack foods in school or college lockers, in a box under the bed at boarding school, in kit bags or in the car for travelling to and from training and matches. Many young players

---

Suitable Snack Food Suggestions

- Cereal, fruit and nut and energy bars – any make or variety
- Jaffa cakes
- Twiglets and pretzels
- Digestive biscuits, ginger nuts, fig rolls
- Jam-filled Swiss rolls, Battenburg cake
- Scones, fruit buns, malt loaf, Scotch pancakes, iced fingers and iced buns (these do not need special storage conditions and have a few days shelf-life)
- Long-life milk shakes that do not need any special storage conditions. (General tip: if the item is on the open shelf in a supermarket it is all right to keep it in a locker or kit bag – though do not leave it close to a radiator)
- Small cartons of fruit juice
- Fresh fruit
- Dried fruit – raisins, apricots, apples, peaches etc.

---

involved in playing not only at school but at clubs or as part of the England Rugby Academy system, often have to travel after school for over an hour to get to training sessions. From lunch-time to the start of training is too long to go without food, so suitable items must be available to eat on the journey. More food will be needed for refuelling after training. Again, this will often be consumed in the car on the way home, although some may be eaten in the changing rooms immediately after training has finished.

Breakfast Habits

Breakfast is perhaps the most important meal of the day as it breaks the fast of the night when most young players will not have eaten anything for eight to twelve hours. It tops up low blood sugar (glucose) levels as well as the stores of carbohydrate (glycogen) in the liver. These will have been used to provide fuel for the brain and other organs, which, thankfully, continue to work while the body sleeps. Generally players cannot afford to miss any meals, but this is particularly true for young players, and missing breakfast will make it difficult for players to meet their daily energy requirements.

Having breakfast reduces the risk of eating unsuitable foods later on the way to school, college or work. It also prevents hunger pangs setting in during lessons or work-time, which will help to maintain concentration levels. The body dehydrates during the night (unless fluids are taken on board during wakeful moments and after nocturnal visits to the loo) and breakfast can start the rehydrating process, too.

What makes a good breakfast? Of course, one that is nutritionally sound, but also one that is enjoyed, particularly for those who need to be encouraged to fall out of bed 15min earlier in order to start getting into the breakfast habit. Parents and guardians should help their young players to start having breakfast if they do not at the moment, perhaps by suggesting they go to bed 15min earlier?

Missing breakfast seems to be a British

habit, and statistics show that the average Briton misses 114 breakfasts a year compared to seventy-two among continental counterparts. It is possible to change breakfast habits, though. Having given a short presentation to a group of thirteen-year-old players in the changing room about the importance of breakfast, the author duly gave them their handouts and sent them on their way. A week later she received an email from a mother which read, 'I am not sure what you said, but my son is now a breakfast convert! I have tried for years to get him to have breakfast – all to no avail. By the way, if you would like to mention that keeping his bedroom tidy and doing his homework will also be beneficial to his rugby performance on the pitch, I would be eternally grateful.'

Lunch

Food-based standards for school lunches (that is, based on specific foods to be included or excluded over the course of a week) were introduced in September 2006 (see Appendix V), and additional nutrient-based standards (that is, setting out the levels of required nutrients, regardless of which foods they are derived from) will be in place in secondary schools from September 2009.

The main problem that young players will meet at lunchtime will be more in terms of the quantity rather than the quality of the food offered. If players feel they are not getting enough to eat and portions cannot be increased, extra food will be needed not just as emergency rations in the locker, but as food supplies taken into school daily, such as sandwiches or filled rolls.

For players at boarding school, problems can occur when fridges have to be shared. Teenage rugby players probably need a small fridge each to store enough extra food such as milk, cheese and yogurts. Dried milk powder and milk-shake syrups could be used if this is not an option – though players must make sure that they wash out the shaker very thoroughly with washing-up liquid and hot water.

Other issues that may need to be addressed include missing meals because of extra train-

---

Eating Schedule for a Player at Day School

The following is the eating schedule for a seventeen-year-old élite player at a day school.

Monday
7.30am Breakfast
10.15am Break: toast and cake
1.30pm School lunch and packed lunch
Refueller straight after school, before training
Refueller straight after training
6.00–9.00pm Dinner
Bedtime: toast or cereal

Tuesday
7.30am Breakfast
10.15am Break: as Monday
1.30pm School lunch and packed lunch
Refueller after school
6.00–9.00pm Dinner
Bedtime: toast or cereal

Wednesday
(Either a match or games in the afternoon)
7.30am Breakfast
10.15am Break: as Monday, plus some of the packed lunch if missing lunch because of a match
1.30pm School lunch before rugby training, and some of the packed lunch
Immediately after training: rest of the packed lunch
OR if no match tea provided: rest of the packed lunch
6.00–9.00pm Dinner
Bedtime: toast or cereal

Thursday
7.30am Breakfast
10.15 Break: as Monday
1.30pm School lunch and packed lunch
Refueller on way to Academy training (fairly long journey)
Refueller on way home from training
Before bed: Baked beans on toast with cheese and glass of milk

Friday
Similar to Tuesday

ing sessions, or because they have to travel to an afternoon match at another school. Such problems can be surmounted, however, they just need some careful planning, perhaps by both school and parents – as the example in the panel shows.

Thursday is a particularly difficult day as it is essential the player arrives at the evening training session not hungry but comfortable enough to do hard training, which involves some weights. Nutritionally the refuellers must therefore provide plenty of carbohydrate for energy, as well as some protein. As dinner is missed, the player needs to make sure that enough fruit and if possible vegetables and salad are eaten during the day.

Top Tips on What to Eat

- Eat regular meals and snacks, including breakfast.
- Young players will need to eat more than their friends who do not exercise very much, if at all.
- Include carbohydrate (bread, breakfast cereals, pasta, rice, noodles or potatoes) in every meal for energy.
- Include protein (meat, chicken, fish, eggs, milk and baked beans) in every meal for muscle growth.
- Aim to have at least five portions of fruit and vegetables every day for general health and growth.
- Refuel as soon as possible after all training sessions (sandwich, banana, milk shake, Jaffa cakes, sports drink).
- Including some sugary sources is probably essential if carbohydrate requirements are to be met.
- Eating late at night is okay (bowl of cereal and banana or toast and jam or honey and a glass of milk): never go to bed hungry.
- Keep a sense of proportion about high fat foods (for example, fast foods, fried foods and pastry) – not never, just not often or frequently.
- Always keep sensible snacks in the school locker or bag so hunger can always be kept at bay.

MATCHES

Information about what to eat and drink around matches has already been covered in Chapter 4, but this may not be so relevant for young school or club teams. As children are the least efficient at regulating body temperature, it is important that they are given the opportunity to drink before the game and during the warm-up.

Drinks should be encouraged during stoppages, and particularly at half-time for all players. Suitable choices are water, squash or a sports drink. Small amounts of fruit such as chunks of banana or orange quarters can also be passed round at half time as the team huddle together discussing how the match is going.

At the end of the match, assorted sandwiches or filled rolls and fruit can be provided to start the refuelling process quickly. If a cooked meal is to be provided, popular and nutritionally balanced suggestions include shepherd's pie with peas/carrots, spaghetti bolognese, fish fingers with mashed potato and peas, fish pie with a mashed potato topping, tuna pasta bake or something as simple as jacket potato with baked beans/tuna/cheese, French bread, cheese and tomato pizza, or baked beans on toast with fruit and/or yogurt to follow.

MENTAL PERFORMANCE

The recommendation to enjoy a diet high in carbohydrate for physical performance can also help young players who must consider mental performance, not just in relation to rugby but also for their studies. The brain is the most active organ in the body, and it needs a steady supply of glucose as its primary source of energy. However, very little glucose is stored in the brain and a constant supply is needed to meet its minimum requirement of about 100g of glucose a day.

The amount of glucose that is used by the brain increases during times of intense concentration. What appears to be particularly important is the effect glucose availability has on tasks that require sustained concentration for longer periods of time. A number of

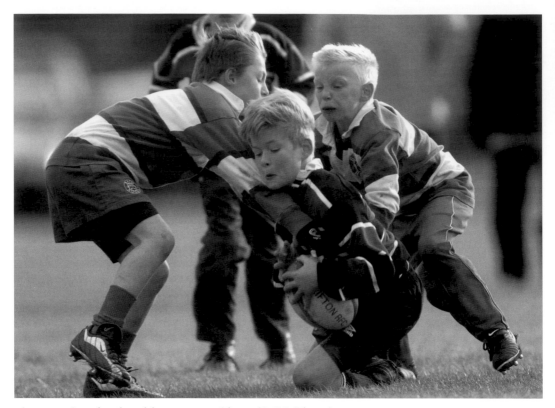

A game of rugby played by a group of boys. (© PA Photos)

scientific studies have been carried out to measure the effect of blood sugar on the brain's performance, and they clearly show the importance of carbohydrate food and snacks to keep the energy supply to the brain topped up. It seems that a carbohydrate-rich snack between meals can boost memory and the performance of mentally demanding tasks. This could help the young player not just with studying, but in rugby training and matches, too.

LIVING AWAY FROM HOME

Young players who can plan weekly menus, shop (usually on a tight budget) and prepare their own meals will find it less of a struggle to achieve the correct diet in terms of quality and quantity in order to maximize both physical and mental performance when they move away from home to college, university or to a club as part of the England Rugby Academy

system. Planning meals on a weekly basis is the best way to budget financially and to minimize the time involved in preparing meals on a regular daily basis.

If players are sharing a house the first thing to decide is if meals are going to be cooked and eaten together, or if everyone is going to be self-sufficient. Sharing can help to keep the costs down, and it also takes away the burden of preparing a cooked meal every day. Most players will probably prefer to cook less often, albeit in larger quantities when they do.

COOKING SKILLS

Players will only need to know how to cook a few basic meals, as one simple meal can often be turned into a number of different meals quite easily. Once a bolognese sauce has been mastered, a player will be able to make spaghetti (or any other pasta) bolognese, chilli con carne with rice or pasta (by just

Budget Cooking

The following are key points when working to a tight budget:

- Decide how much is to be spent on food.
- Keep a list in the kitchen to note down when items are running low.
- Keep to the shopping list, and avoid impulse buying in the supermarket.
- Do not over-shop, particularly if there is limited storage available.
- Buy all the dry goods (pasta, rice, breakfast cereals etc.) for the week, and some perishables (fruit and vegetables). Buy more perishables later in the week. That way no food will end up being thrown away because it has gone off.
- Check if local greengrocers and butchers are cheaper than the supermarket.
- Look out for special offers, such as 'two for the price of one'. However, these are only bargains if they would have been bought anyway.
- Buying 'own brand' items is often cheaper (supermarket label breakfast cereals instead of 'well-known' names). This is not always true, so prices should be checked, especially on a weight basis.
- Storing food correctly means money will not be wasted should rotten food have to be thrown away.
- Put food in and out of the fridge quickly. Opening the door warms up the interior temperature, as does putting warm food straight into the fridge. This can speed up food going off.
- Check for forgotten foods at the back of the fridge. Do not let the smell be the reminder.
- Clean the fridge and defrost the freezer regularly as this helps to keep them running efficiently and effectively. Check the instruction book on how to do this.

adding a can of red kidney beans and chilli powder to taste) or shepherd's pie (by boiling and mashing potatoes). Even simpler, frozen peas can be cooked in the sauce and then served on toast or warmed pitta breads, or on top of a jacket potato or two.

Having learnt how to cut up meat into small bite-sized pieces and to prepare vegetables (or buy a bag of stir-fry vegetables), a player can make a variety of different stir-fry dishes using chicken, turkey, pork, lamb or beef. Even canned tuna can work. Again this can be served with noodles, pasta or rice.

Grilling meats, bacon and fish is much better nutritionally than traditional frying, as the fat drips out into the grill pan underneath. It is an easy and quick method of cooking, though it is important to get the heat and timing right. The down side of grilling is cleaning the grill pan afterwards. Letting the fat cool down a little, then pouring it into an old mug to solidify is probably the easiest option. The grill pan can then be washed out with hot soapy water.

CHAPTER 9
Injury and Illness

At the élite end of the game the number of injuries in English rugby union is close to 1,500 a season. A large-scale study of match injuries sustained by professional rugby union players concluded that on average, a club has 18 per cent of their players unavailable for selection as a consequence of match injuries. (*See* References Chapter 9, 1.) The same study found that on average, a club has 5 per cent of their players unavailable for selection as a result of training injuries. (*See* References Chapter 9, 2.) Training injuries tended to be towards the beginning of the season, with one-third of all training injuries recorded as a result of pre-season training.

Putting match and training injuries together, 23 per cent of an average club's squad are likely to be unavailable for selection at any one time. Forwards and backs most commonly sustained thigh haematomas (swellings caused by the accumulation of clotted blood in tissues), and the longest absences from play were, for forwards, as a result of anterior cruciate damage, and for backs, hamstring injuries. Rucks and mauls caused the most injuries to forwards, and being tackled caused most injuries to backs. At greatest risk of injury are hookers and the outside centre.

A prospective study of injuries to the England rugby union players during preparation for and participation in the 2003 Rugby World Cup found that the tackle, ruck and maul elements of match play, and the endurance running and contact elements of training, presented the highest risk of injury for all players. (*See* References Chapter 9, 3.) An Australian study undertaken in the 2002 and 2003 seasons identified the risk and patterns of injury across multiple levels in rugby union from Under-15 schoolboy teams to the Australian national team. For known events, tackling was the main cause of injury, causing a third of all injuries. Musculoskeletal injury accounted for the majority of missed games in rugby, with more serious injuries in the older players, and a higher rate of concussion in younger players.

An earlier study examined the influence of training and match intensity, duration and load on the incidence of injury over the course of a season in rugby league players (*see* References Chapter 9, 4). These researchers suggested that as the intensity, duration and load of rugby league training sessions and matches increased, the incidence of injury also increased. With such statistics, players and coaches will want to know if diet can help in speeding up recovery time from injuries.

DIET AND THE HEALING PROCESS

It has long been known that adequate amounts of protein, vitamins and minerals are needed for the healing process, and that inadequate amounts can delay the process or lead to poor healing. However, it is important to take into account changes in energy requirements, particularly if an extended lay-off is envisaged. Injured players may not automatically reduce their food intake because of the drop in physical activity level – indeed, intakes may not change very much if boredom-eating sets in. A simple way to cut back portion sizes is to use a slightly smaller bowl and plate from usual: even piling these up as much as the usual larger bowl and plate will automatically reduce intake.

Breaks for treatment and rehabilitation of injuries can lead to deconditioning and a risk of increase in body fat and a decrease in muscle mass. This can slow the process of rehabilitation and return to form. Muscle mass will be lost if weights sessions have to be stopped or surgery requires parts of the body to be immobilized. A bulking-up diet may therefore be needed at some stage during the rehabilitation programme. However, it is important not to cut back intake drastically as the recovery process itself does increase requirements – just not as much as the decrease due to the cutback in training and match play. An unnecessarily vicious restriction on food intake can certainly slow recovery. Most players will find they need to reduce their intake of carbohydrate because their requirements are lower, which will help to reduce the overall energy intake. Protein intake should not be reduced, but neither should fat intake be increased.

MUSCLE INJURIES

Much of the swelling and soreness following a muscle injury comes from an increase in free radicals: it is therefore important to increase dietary intake of antioxidants to mop these up. This involves ensuring that plenty of fruits and vegetables are eaten on a daily basis – and the more varied the colours, the wider the range of antioxidants that will be consumed. Vitamin C is a powerful antioxidant, so including some orange juice with breakfast every day would be helpful.

Fruit and vegetables provide more than just the antioxidant vitamins and minerals: they also contain thousands of phytochemicals – different ones in different fruits and vegetables. So reaching for the multivitamin and mineral pill is not the answer.

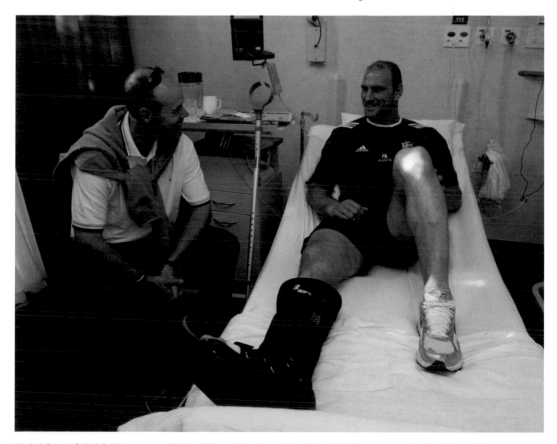

British and Irish Lions coach Sir Clive Woodward talks with Lawrence Dallaglio as he rests his broken ankle in Auckland (2005). (© PA Photos)

Damage to muscles results in a breakdown of muscle proteins, so these need to be replaced by protein from the diet. There should be no need to buy, or to continue to use, expensive protein supplements: just make sure that each meal contains good quality protein such as lean meat, chicken, white and oily fish, eggs and milk. Protein-rich food from animal sources contains proteins that are more like those in our bodies. However, vegetable sources such as pulses, nuts and seeds can be used to top-up intakes.

Zinc is a mineral that may also help recovery; a good source is lean meat. Clams and oysters are excellent sources, but not usually foods that are included in the regular daily diet.

Creatine supplementation has been shown to help the recovery of muscle volume and muscular functional capacity during rehabilitation training after muscle atrophy due to a limb being immobilized. This may be an option worth considering if it could help post-injury rehabilitation, and perhaps return a player back to training and match play. (*See* References Chapter 9, 5.)

A Word about Alcohol

Standard medical practice is to treat soft tissue damage with vasoconstriction or RICE techniques (rest, ice, compression and elevation). Alcohol, on the other hand, is a very good vasodilator, particularly of the blood vessels to the skin, and it has been suggested that excessive amounts of alcohol might lead to further swelling at the injury site, and a slow recovery. Though this has not been shown experimentally, anecdotal evidence suggests that sensible advice is to avoid alcohol, certainly in the first twenty-four hours after the injury. Players facing a long lay-off through injury may be tempted to drink more alcohol than they usually drink when they are fully fit. This may well lead to unwelcome weight gain.

FRACTURES

Although there may be a need to reduce energy intake, it is also important to ensure that adequate amounts of protein, iron, zinc, calcium and vitamin C are consumed, as these all have a part to play in the healing process. Calcium is the number-one nutrient in terms of bone growth and maintenance, and therefore vital if the injury involves a fracture. Milk is an excellent source of calcium, and even non-milk lovers should try to include some each day, perhaps by disguising it as custard or cheese sauce, or using milk rather than water to make porridge. Milk is not the only source of calcium: even dairy ice-cream provides a useful amount.

Other nutrients and minerals involved in bone health include protein, vitamin C, magnesium and zinc. (Chapter 1 provides information about the best sources of these bone-healing nutrients.)

The Special Case of the Fractured Jaw

Initially a player with a fractured jaw will need to rely solely on whole liquid meals such as Build-up or Complan, which can be made up using full fat, semi-skimmed or skimmed milk. Muscle wastage while unable to train is more likely than an increase in body fat, and a determined effort will be needed to keep up the calorie and protein intake. The sheer volume of fluid needed to maintain energy intake will be quite difficult to achieve, particularly at the beginning, and full fat milk will be the best choice initially. However, this is not an excuse to start loading with double cream…!

These complete products come in a variety of sweet, plain or savoury flavours. The plain variety can be flavoured with a favourite milkshake syrup. These liquid meals will provide carbohydrate, protein, a little fat and vitamins and minerals. Other items that can be introduced immediately, or fairly soon, include full fat milk, protein drinks, puréed bananas, puréed porridge made with milk and sugar, fruit juices (though they may be too acidic at this stage), milky tea, coffee or hot chocolate and squash. The aim is to include items that will contribute a good range of nutrients or that are going to contribute to keeping the body hydrated. Oral hygiene is very important, as protein and energy-containing fluids are an ideal medium for bacterial growth: so regular use of a suitable mouthwash is essential.

As things begin to settle down it should be possible to start introducing home-made or bought fresh soups such as carrot and coriander, leek and potato, tomato with basil and pumpkin, puréed if necessary, and smoothies made with milk, yogurt and fresh fruit.

The next step will be to introduce soft foods that do not require chewing but which have more texture or are thicker. Suitable items include fruit purées, custard, yogurt and fromage frais, ice cream, mousses and fruit fools. Mashed or puréed potatoes flavoured with herbs, tomato or garlic purée, mustard or a little olive oil can bring a welcome variation. Melting some grated cheese or low fat soft cheese into the potatoes adds protein, calcium and other minerals and vitamins as well as flavour. To relieve the boredom, carrots, sweet potato, pumpkin, swede or turnip can all be mashed or puréed too.

Finally before getting back to enjoying a full diet the following should be manageable – canned baked beans (though the skins may be difficult), canned pasta shapes in tomato or cheese sauce, canned lentils flavoured with a little curry powder (imagine it is a dhal curry), canned rice pudding with jam, flaked canned tuna or salmon softened with a little lemon juice or mayonnaise, scrambled egg, wheat biscuits with plenty of milk as a change from porridge, and cooked fresh fish (flaked and all bones removed and mixed with a white sauce flavoured with cheese). At the last stage before getting back to normal meals again, minced meats, bread and rice can be introduced.

It may be difficult for some players to maintain their diet while they are injured. Food shopping may be difficult because of reduced mobility, or cooking may be awkward if only one hand is operational. This is when family, friends, housemates and girlfriends can be very helpful!

MUSCLE CRAMPS

Muscle cramps occur most often in the calf, hamstrings and quadriceps. They can last seconds or minutes, and cause anything from a twinge to excruciating pain for a player. The muscle contracts involuntarily and does not relax due probably to abnormal stimulation. Why this should happen remains a mystery. Cramps tend to occur in tired muscles – hence they are usually seen in the later stages of matches or hard training sessions.

Possible causes include dehydration, where there are high fluid and sodium losses, but depletion of other minerals seems less likely. Creatine usage has been implicated by some people, but again this seems unlikely. Studies have not found any difference in the prevalence of cramps in creatine users and non-users. Cramps also tend to occur more often with increasing age.

How to Avoid Cramps

- Drink plenty of fluids to avoid dehydration.
- Consider using a sports drink, particularly if a heavy salt sweater.
- Increase strength and fitness so fatigue is delayed. Cramps are less common in well-trained individuals.
- Be careful when changing speed or intensity towards the end of training and matches. Adapting to an increased workload takes longer when muscles are tired.
- Ensure clothing and footwear are comfortable and not too tight.
- Consider adding salt to the post-training or post-match meal.
- Rest thoroughly after hard training sessions.
- If cramp does occur – stretch, massage the muscle and hydrate using a sports drink.

HEAT CRAMPS

The association between heat cramps and sodium levels is not new. For over a century, stokers on ocean steamers, miners, desert soldiers and workers labouring during hot summer months have learned the importance of adding salt to their drinks to help prevent cramping. Rugby is turning into an all-the-year-round sport, particularly when pre-season training and summer tours are taken into account. As players experience warmer weather at the beginning and end of the season, together with greater sweat loss than normal, heat cramps may become a fairly common occurrence.

Heat cramps are caused by an imbalance in the body's fluid volume and electrolyte concentration, together with low energy stores. The core temperature, however, remains in the normal range. Magnesium, potassium and calcium deficiencies have all been suggested, but loss of these minerals in sweat is negligible. Many researchers believe the cause is sodium depletion. Heat cramps appear to occur in heavy sweaters who produce particularly salty sweat. This shows as salt caked on the skin or as white marks on clothing, particularly around the armpits and groin – very obvious when players are wearing black kit. Non-crampers tend not to sweat as much or to lose as much salt in their sweat as crampers.

Players prone to heat cramps should use a sports drink rather than water, and should eat salty snacks such as pretzels and crackers. The general advice to reduce salt intake is aimed very much at the inactive, overweight/obese section of the population, rather than the very physically active. Players in doubt about adding salt to their diet (perhaps where there is a family history of high blood pressure, for example) should talk to their GP.

THE STITCH

The stitch seems to be much less common amongst rugby players than muscle cramps, but it does still happen during certain types of training, mostly notably and not surprisingly when running. Scientists have been puzzled for some time about what causes the stitch. A possible cause was thought to be lack of oxygen resulting from a reduction in blood supply to the diaphragm as blood was directed away to the exercising muscles. Others have thought it was just the effect of food and fluid in the small intestine pulling on the ligaments attached to the diaphragm.

The favoured theory is that the stitch is caused by the two layers of membranes in the abdominal area (one attached to the abdominal wall and the other covering the organs in the abdomen, namely the stomach, liver and spleen) rubbing against each other. The layers are separated by lubricating fluid, and it is believed that friction could arise because of a distended stomach, or because dehydration has reduced the amount of lubricating fluid, or even just because of an overall increased movement in the area through running. Apart from easing off and dropping the exercise intensity (which may not always be possible), bending forwards, pushing the painful spot and breathing deeply can bring relief.

How to Avoid a Stitch

- Allow between two and four hours between a meal and hard training or a match, if prone to getting a stitch.
- Avoid high fat foods as they take longer to digest.
- Make pre-exercise meals high carbohydrate, moderate-to-low protein, and low fat.
- Be well hydrated before training and matches.
- Take all opportunities to drink during training and matches so that regular, small amounts maintain hydration.
- Avoid drinking infrequently, and then needing to drink a large volume of fluid.
- Avoid hypertonic drinks (fruit juice, soft drinks and hypertonic energy drinks) during training and matches, as they empty slowly from the stomach and could cause distension and increase the risk of a stitch.
- Sports drinks and water are the best choices as they empty quickly from the stomach.

GUT PROBLEMS

Constipation is uncommon in athletes, and rugby players are no exception. This is because regular exercise helps to keep the bowel in good working order. On the other hand, diarrhoea is more common, in some cases due to poor hygiene in the kitchen and bathroom, but mainly due to pre-match nerves. In hard exercise the blood supply to the intestine is reduced so that more blood can be directed to the exercising muscles. This means the digestive powers of the intestine become less efficient. Dehydration, accompanied by the reduced blood supply, can cause the gut to go into spasm, resulting in diarrhoea. Pre-match food intake may not be ideal, which could also contribute to the problem (*see* Chapter 4).

If attention to a sensible match strategy for food and fluid intake does not improve the situation, taking a dose of Imodium (Ioperimide) should help to control things. However, if symptoms get worse or occur more often, advice should be sought from the GP or club doctor.

THE IMMUNE SYSTEM

A healthy immune system is crucial to a rugby player as it is involved in repairing tissues after injury and in protecting the body against potentially damaging bacteria, viruses and fungi. The immune system is a network of physical barriers (skin and tissues in the lungs, nose and intestinal tract), chemical barriers (pH of body fluids such as the acidity in the stomach) and phagocytic cells (cells that can engulf and digest foreign or other particles or cells harmful to the body).

Strenuous exercise can act as a stressor, which can temporarily depress the immune system, but this is usually reversed with rest. However, the stress response is likely to be exacerbated if a player has a poor diet, is not sleeping well, or is under some psychological stress. Unfamiliar surroundings such as being away from home can also intensify the stress response. This could apply to a foreign player joining a club. Diet might be poor because he is unfamiliar with the food and shops, and the strange surroundings may be affecting his sleep pattern. The resulting stress response may manifest itself in an increased incidence of upper respiratory tract infections.

The main culprit is the stress hormone cortisol, which is released when heavy bouts of exercise are performed. Though it does help the body to turn fat and protein into sources of energy that it can use when supplies of glucose are low, it does have a down side, too, in that it suppresses phagocytes, which destroy invading organisms in the blood, and IgA, an antibody found in saliva. This suppression of the immune system continues for a number of hours after intense exercise.

Research at Loughborough University has shown that the immune suppression is much lower if a sports drink is consumed at the rate of a litre an hour during a run. Consuming more carbohydrate keeps the blood glucose level more stable so the body does not need to use fat and protein as fuel, resulting in less cortisol being released.

Probiotics are believed to help fight illness by improving the balance of bacteria in the gut. Researchers in Australia tested this theory out using well-trained recreational athletes. Nine athletes had referred themselves to a medical sports clinic complaining of fatigue, recurrent sore throats and impaired performance. Eighteen athletes acted as a healthy control group. After taking a four-week course of the probiotic supplement *L. acidophilus*, not only did the fatigued athletes show signs of improved immune function at the end of the study, but the healthy group did, too. (*See* References Chapter 9, 6.)

COLD CURES

For those players unlucky enough to succumb to a cold there are actions they can take that may minimize the number of days they feel grotty. General advice is to keep up fluid intake, eat lots of fruit and vegetables, try to rest as much as possible, and take paracetamol or aspirin to ease the symptoms. Vitamin C may also help to lessen the severity and the number of days the cold is hanging about. Take a dose of 500–1,000mg vitamin C every day from the first sign of a cold, and continue until it has gone. This is not recommended as a prophylactic – there is no evidence that it stops a cold, just that it eases symptoms once a cold has been caught.

Zinc lozenges are commonly used as prophylactics against the common cold. Since 1984, eleven studies have been carried out on zinc supplements in the treatment of the common cold, and five reported beneficial effects and six did not. However, to be effective in reducing the duration or severity of

Practical Ways to Reduce Risk of Infection

- Ensure adequate rest after all training to allow time for adaptations to occur. Include one or two rest days each week. Training is the stimulus to which the body adapts, but rest time is needed to allow adaptations to take place.
- Eat well. Ensure adequate energy intake in relation to training load. Make sure the diet contains plenty of fruit and vegetables, and good quality protein-rich foods. The more colourful fruits and vegetables tend to have the highest levels of antioxidants.
- A broad-spectrum multivitamin and mineral supplement can be beneficial to top up dietary intakes that may not always be optimal, but megadosing should be avoided as this can be counter-productive.
- Consider using a probiotic.
- Get adequate sleep (around six to eight hours). Sleep quality is also important, so keep to a regular pattern, going to bed and getting up at roughly the same time every day.
- Do not share drinks bottles, cutlery or food with others, especially team-mates, as this is one way infections are passed on.
- Reduce exposure to infection by bacteria and viruses by washing hands after using the toilet and before meals.
- Keep hands away from the eyes and mouth.
- Cover the nose with a scarf in cold weather when practical. Viruses multiply in the lining of the nose, and they breed faster when the cells are cool.
- Avoid dehydration and getting a dry mouth. Drink regularly during training and matches. Saliva contains antibacterial proteins, but saliva flow tends to fall during exercise.
- Use a sports drink, as the carbohydrate in the drink helps maintain immune function. This is particularly important in long (90-plus minutes) or very intense training sessions, and of course matches.
- Keeping a log of mood, perceptions of difficulty in training, feelings of fatigue and muscle soreness, can help to indicate unusual tiredness.
- Make some lifestyle changes to include mental relaxation and stress management strategies. Mental stress is closely related to overtraining, and can lead to an increased risk of upper respiratory tract infections.
- Avoid contact with people with colds, flu or infections – particularly straight after training and matches, as there is an increased susceptibility to infection in the first few hours after finishing.
- Consider a flu injection, particularly for those susceptible or at high risk of infection, such as teachers.
- Reduce the intensity and duration of training, or skip altogether if symptoms of illness are present.
- If symptoms of illness are above the neck (dry, sore throat, blocked or runny nose, sneezing, slightly swollen glands), undertake light exercise until the symptoms have gone, and then gradually build up to full training.
- Skip training if symptoms are below the neck (productive cough, general aches and pains, fever, overwhelming tiredness or fatigue, rise in heart rate (+20 per cent)). See a doctor and take advice about when to resume training.

cold symptoms, the supplement must be taken within twenty-four hours of symptom onset. If there is no clear improvement within three days, supplementation should be discontinued.

Echinacea is another possibility. There have been conflicting views on its benefits in the past, but new research showing how and why we suffer cold symptoms has thrown light on the beneficial effects. The cold virus does not invade the whole body, and then cause various unpleasant symptoms: it actually stays in the lining of the nose and upper part of the respiratory tract where it reproduces, and it is the reproduction of the virus and the body's immune reaction to it that causes the feelings usually associated with a cold. It is believed the echinacea calms the immune system, prevents this reaction, and so keeps symptoms at bay. Evidence for efficacy supports only fresh extracts of *Echinacea purpurea*, ideally in tincture form.

Garlic and chillies appear to help minimize cold effects for some people, while others find relief by adding a few drops of eucalyptus oil to a bowl of steaming water, covering the head with a towel, and inhaling the steam deeply. This last remedy may not appeal to everybody, and may certainly depend on their living situation.

JOINT CARE

Arthritis is a term that covers a number of conditions characterized by inflammation of the joints. The most common is osteoarthritis (OA), which results from degeneration and wearing away of the cartilage (gristle), which normally acts as a shock absorber, cushioning the bones and providing a smooth surface for the bones to slide against. If the cartilage becomes thinner and rougher, the bones start to grind against each other causing pain, inflammation, stiffness and impaired movement. It is more common in sportsmen and women than the general population, and occurs particularly in those who take part in high impact sports, which of course includes rugby. Osteoarthritis of the knee poses a significant risk to serious rugby players, particularly amongst those who sustain knee injuries during their playing careers.

Omega-3 fatty acids may help to slow the destruction of joint cartilage in players with OA. Studies certainly look promising. In a small study, thirty-one OA patients were randomized to receive two capsules a day containing 1,000mg cod liver oil (a rich source of omega-3 fatty acids) or a placebo oil. (*See* References Chapter 9, 7.) The results of the study implied that ingestion of omega-3 fatty acids may impede disease progression by stopping or slowing cartilage degeneration in OA patients. This is particularly encouraging for players who have suffered sporting injuries that predispose to early onset of OA. Advice to such players would be to consider taking cod liver oil at this level of supplementation to help prevent further joint damage.

Glucosamine and chondroitin, both components of cartilage and connective tissue, are two other supplements promoted for joint health, and specifically in the treatment of OA. As its name suggests, glucosamine is formed from glucose and the amino acid glutamine. Found predominantly in cartilage, its function is to keep the cartilage healthy and resilient. It is thought that joint cartilage is constantly being rebuilt and that worn-out or damaged cartilage is therefore replaced. Glucosamine has been shown to help in this regeneration of cartilage as well as having anti-inflammatory properties. The majority of studies have shown that regular supplementation with glucosamine offers some pain relief and improved function in people who have regular knee pain. It usually takes six weeks of regular supplementation for the beneficial effects to become noticeable. Chondroitin's function is to draw fluid and nutrients into cartilage tissue. The fluid acts rather like a spongy shock absorber, helping to protect cartilage from premature breakdown.

The Glucosamine/chondroitin Arthritis Intervention Trial (GAIT) was a long-awaited multi-centre, double-blind trial set up to assess short-term effectiveness (twenty-four weeks) on pain and joint function. (*See* References Chapter 9, 8.) The conclusion from the study, published in 2006, was that glucosamine and chondroitin in combination were effective in treating moderate to severe pain in OA, but not mild pain. The authors suggest this lack of response may be due to a floor effect that limits the ability to detect response.

So should players use these supplements as a prophylactic, to help prevent joint pain and the development of OA? At the moment there is no evidence to suggest they prevent OA or joint pain in healthy players. Indeed, the majority of studies have been undertaken

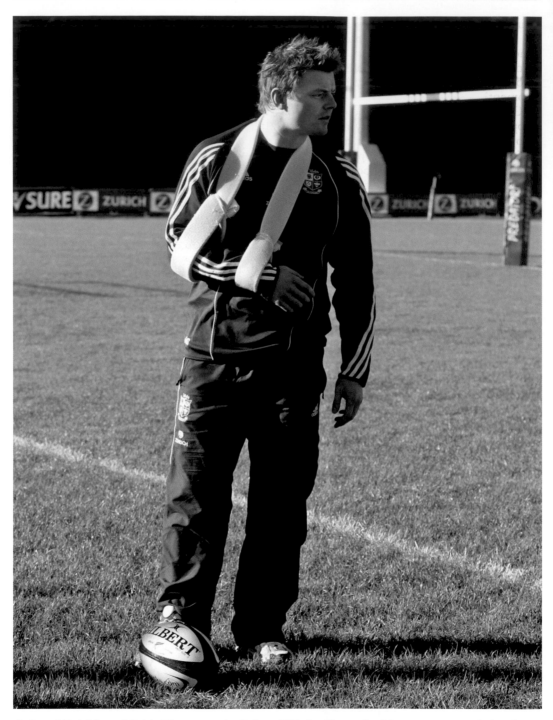

Injured British and Irish Lions captain Brian O'Driscoll watches his tem-mates training in New Zealand. (© PA Photos)

using older people, and applying these results to players may not be appropriate. Players who have suffered a knee injury should certainly consider taking a supplement, but what about players who have healthy joints at the moment?

Glucosamine, chondroitin and cod liver oil supplements are widely used by many sports people, mostly notably distance runners who believe that they do help to preserve joints and keep them working properly and painlessly. Given the high incidence of knee injuries among rugby players it does seem sensible to consider taking a daily joint care supplement. A daily dosage of 1,500mg of glucosamine a day is normally recommended – though care should be taken when selecting a glucosamine supplement. The product must contain enough of the active ingredient (glucosamine sulphate) in the manufacturer's recommended daily dosage. As with any supplementation, it is always recommended that players first get the supplement checked out by a doctor, physiotherapist, sports dietitian, registered performance nutritionist or pharmacist before parting with any money. Any supplement used, for whatever purpose, must be safe and effective, and must not produce a positive drug test (*see* Chapter 7).

Appendices

Ideas for food suitable for the cupboard, fridge and freezer.

Store-Cupboard

Cereal-based foods
- Breakfast cereals – great snack foods, not just for eating at breakfast time
- Pasta – all shapes and sizes; combine with other store-cupboard ingredients to make salads
- Canned spaghetti and ravioli
- Noodles
- Rice – with sauces, in risottos and salads
- Savoury rice
- Instant mashed potatoes
- Grains – cous cous, bulgar wheat, polenta
- Oat cakes, crispbreads and digestive biscuits with cheese, honey, jam or Marmite, etc, for snacking
- Cereal bars
- Pizza base – good standby, add toppings of choice
- Bread sticks, crispbreads, water biscuits, Matzos, etc

Fruit and vegetables
- Canned tomatoes (chopped and passata, with or without herbs) – good for sauces and pizza toppings
- Tomato puree
- Canned beans – baked beans, red kidney beans, butter beans, chilli beans, borlotti beans, cannellini beans and chickpeas; add to sauces, salads, soups or mix with vegetables ti fill pitta pockets
- Canned sweetcorn – mix with baked beans, in a salad or serve as a vegetable

- Canned fruit – a good standby if you run out of fresh fruit (buy the fruit canned in natural juices)
- Canned pineapple mixed with low fat soft cheese makes healthy filling for jacket potatoes
- Dried fruit – raisins sultanas, apricots, dried figs and prunes; for snacking or adding to breakfast cereals or sandwich fillings
- Lemon juice – for flavouring and added vitamin C

Fish
- Canned fish – tuna, sardines, salmon, mackerel and pilchards; for sauces, salads, on toast, in pitta bread pockets or as fillings for jacket potatoes

Dairy produce
- UHT semi-skimmed milk in cartons – useful standby
- Dried skimmed or semi-skimmed milk – another standby

Drinks
- Long-life cartons of fruit juice
- Regular or low-calorie squash or high juice drinks
- Regular or low-calorie fizzy drinks
- Tea, coffee, hot chocolate
- Bottled water

Miscellaneous
- Crunchy or smooth peanut butter
- Marmite, honey, jam and marmalade – for sandwich fillings or toast
- Pasta and stir-fry sauces
- Nuts, fruit and nuts, seeds – for snacks, salads and sauces for pasta and rice
- Canned soups

- Canned condensed soups – double as sauces
- Canned low fat milk puddings – quick, healthy filling pudding
- Canned, cartons or pots of custard
- Instant whips
- Worcestershire sauce – for flavour
- Flour
- Mustards, horseradish sauce, soy sauce, vinegars
- Mint sauce
- Chilli powder, curry powder, dried herbs

Fridge

Cereal-based foods
- Fresh pasta – for example, ravioli: just cook and top with a little Parmesan cheese

Meat and alternatives
- Wafer-thin ham and smoked turkey: good for sandwich fillings or shredding to add to sauces
- Low-fat liver pâté, for sandwiches
- Eggs
- Quorn and tofu – easy and quick to cook with – stir-fry, meat-free bolognese etc.

Dairy produce
- Semi-skimmed milk
- Yogurt – low fat fruit or natural yogurt
- Fromage frais
- Parmesan cheese – useful for toppings on lots of dishes. Long shelf-life
- Low fat soft cheese – for sandwiches, spreading on pitta bread or melting down for sauces
- Cheese

Spreads
- Low fat spread, polyunsaturated margarine or butter

Freezer

Cereal-based foods
- Spare loaves of bread (can be toasted from frozen), rolls, baps and muffins
- Pitta bread: can be heated up in the toaster or under the grill in moments
- Fruit buns, teacakes and scones. Ideal for the kit bag as they thaw out while out training, etc.

- Pizzas and pizza bases
- Waffles
- Low fat Beefeater oven chips

Meat and alternatives
- Lean mince – for meat sauces and cottage/shepherd's pie. Frozen in portions
- Lean cubed meat, for kebabs. Again, frozen in portions
- Low fat sausages and burgers
- Chicken or turkey fillets – grill or for kebabs or cooking in a sauce
- Chicken drumsticks
- Chicken nuggets
- Fish fingers and fish cakes
- Fish steaks

Fruit and vegetables
All frozen vegetables – nutritionally they are just as good as fresh if they are cooked properly.

Dairy produce
- Grated cheese
- Ice cream

APPENDIX II: UNDERSTANDING FOOD LABELS

Sell by (Display by) Dates

These are used by some shops to help staff know when they need to take food products off the shelves. It is not against the law to sell food after this date. However, shops must not sell foods that have passed their 'use by' date.

'Use by' Dates

Shops must not sell foods that have passed their 'use by' date because they might not be safe to eat. 'Use by' dates are used on foods that could go off quickly, for example milk, soft cheese, ready-prepared salads and smoked fish. Even if it looks and smells fine, using it after this date could put health at risk and cause food poisoning. It is important to follow storage instructions given on labels, otherwise the shelf-life of the food could be even shorter than the 'use by' date. Usually food with a 'use by' label needs to be kept in the fridge.

Some food labels also give instructions such as 'eat within a week of opening' and it is important to follow these instructions. But if the 'use by date' is tomorrow, then you must use the food by the end of tomorrow, even if the label says 'eat within a week of opening' and you have only opened the food today.

'Best Before' Dates

These appear on foods that last longer, such as frozen, dried or canned foods. Shops are allowed to sell foods after their 'best before' date, and they will probably be safe to eat. However, remember that if you eat these foods *after* their 'best before' date they might not be as nice to eat as they were before that date. For instance, they might have started to lose their flavour or texture.

Eggs are the one food you should *not* eat after its 'best before' date, because eggs can contain salmonella bacteria, which could start to multiply after this date.

APPENDIX III: FOOD SAFETY

Improper handling and storage of food and leftovers is one of the most common causes of food poisoning in the home. Training schedules and matches can be seriously disrupted by a bout of food poisoning, which can spread if players share a house together. Here are a few simple guidelines to help players avoid an upset tummy.

Storing Food

- Raw meat and poultry must not come into contact with cooked or ready-to-eat food. Drips from raw food must not fall on other food, including food in the salad drawer at the bottom of the fridge.
- Uncooked foods should be on the lowest shelf in the fridge.
- Cooked and uncooked food should never be on the same shelf.
- Left-overs should be cooled quickly in a shallow dish, covered and then put into the fridge or freezer within two hours. Putting hot food into the fridge causes a rise in temperature and encourages condensation and possible contamination of other foods.
- As a general rule, leftovers kept in the fridge should be eaten within two days.
- Hot foods should be kept hot, and cold foods cold: they should not be just left lying around.
- Cooked food should only be reheated once, whether cooked in the kitchen or bought as a cook-chill product. Any leftovers after reheating must be thrown away.
- Left-over canned food should be emptied into a bowl or plastic container (not left in the can), covered and stored in the fridge.

Handling and Preparing Food

- Hands must be clean when handling food, and washed between handling raw foods and cooked or ready-to-eat foods.
- Knives and other kitchen utensils should also be washed between handling raw and cooked foods.
- Working surfaces should be washed frequently and thoroughly.
- Particular attention should be paid to washing chopping boards.
- Cooked or ready-to-eat food should not be placed on a surface that has just had raw food on it.
- Vegetables, salads and fruits should be washed in clean, cold, running water.
- If using dried beans, including red kidney beans, the beans must be soaked in water for up to twelve hours (or overnight), the water thrown away and the beans then boiled briskly in fresh water for at least 10min to destroy the toxins in the raw beans. Canned beans can be used straight from the can as the canning process destroys the toxins.

Thawing and Cooking Food

- Thawing and cooking instructions on frozen foods should be read and followed carefully. Meat and poultry must be completely thawed before cooking.
- After thawing frozen poultry there should be no ice particles and the flesh should be soft and pliable.

- Food should be cooked well; the instructions on the pack should always be followed.
- When food is reheated it should be heated until piping hot.

What Not to Eat

Leftovers of questionable age and safety should never be tasted. If a leftover has been stored for too long, or looks or smells peculiar, it must be thrown away.

Personal Hygiene

- Hands should be washed after going to the toilet and after handling pets.
- Domestic pets should be kept out of the kitchen if possible, but certainly away from food, dishes and worktops.

APPENDIX IV: MEAL IDEAS

Breakfast

- Cereals, any variety including porridge
- Fruit – any, but especially bananas and dried fruit
- Toast, rolls, English muffins, bagels, crumpets, Scotch pancakes, currant buns
- Low fat spread, butter or margarine
- Jam, honey, marmalade, peanut butter, golden syrup, maple syrup, Marmite or Vegemite
- Low fat soft cheese
- Fruit juice
- Milk, yogurt, milk shakes, smoothies
- Tea, coffee, hot chocolate, squash, water
- Grilled tomatoes
- Poached mushrooms
- Baked beans
- Lean grilled bacon
- Boiled, scrambled or poached eggs
- Omelettes
- Fish fingers
- Potato cakes
- Cold meats and cheese
- Pancakes

Quick Meals and Snacks

- Baked beans or spaghetti in tomato sauce

on toast or pitta bread (add grated cheese for extra protein)
- Lentil, thick vegetable or minestrone soups with bread, toast or pitta bread
- Toasted muffins with low fat soft cheese
- Pitta bread with houmous
- Jacket potato (cooked in the microwave) with baked beans or tuna and sweetcorn
- 'Halfway pizza': warm pitta bread under the grill, spread with tomato sauce (not ketchup), sprinkle with canned, drained sweetcorn, top with grated cheese, and warm again under the grill until the cheese melts
- Omelettes filled with cheese, or cooked frozen vegetables, canned sweetcorn and tuna, cooked chicken or ham, and eaten with chunks of bread
- Scrambled eggs and sweetcorn on toast or muffins
- Pasta with a quick sauce made with chopped onions, canned tomatoes, garlic and herbs. Top with grated cheese, Parmesan cheese or tuna
- Breakfast cereal with milk, chopped banana and extra dried fruit, nuts and seeds
- Sandwiches made with different breads (baguettes, rolls, bagels) and different fillings (turkey and cranberry sauce; ham, cheese and pickle; tuna and sweetcorn; lean bacon, lettuce and tomato; peanut butter and jam)
- Finish with fresh fruit, cereal bar, cake, yogurt and a drink

Main Meal Ideas

Cooked mince meals
- Spaghetti bolognaise made with lean mince, onions, canned chopped tomatoes, tomato purée and herbs
- Chilli con carne as above, but add canned red kidney beans and chilli, and serve with boiled rice
- Shepherd's pie/cottage pie made as for spaghetti bolognaise, top with cooked mashed potato, and serve with peas and carrots

Cooked chicken meals
- Roast chicken with boiled, roast or jacket potatoes and vegetables

- Chicken stir-fry with vegetables and noodles
- Chicken pieces cooked with onions and canned chopped tomatoes and herbs, and served with pasta
- Chicken pieces cooked with onions, with a low fat soft cheese added just before serving to make a sauce, and served with pasta and peas
- Chicken curry with rice (using a ready-made sauce and extra vegetables)

Meat meals
- Stir-fry lean beef or pork pieces with vegetables. Serve with rice or noodles
- Grilled lean meat with mashed or boiled potatoes and vegetables

Fish meals
- Pasta with tomato sauce and tuna
- Tuna pasta bake
- Grilled fish or fish fingers with mashed potato and vegetables and a bought sauce (e.g. parsley, mushroom or white wine)
- Couscous, salmon pieces and cooked peas all mixed together and served with a bought (or home-made) honey and mustard sauce

Vegetarian meals
- Vegetable or lentil curry with rice (using a ready-made sauce and extra vegetables)
- Macaroni cheese with grilled tomatoes
- Deep-pan pizza with tomatoes, sweetcorn and cheese

Puddings
- Pancakes with golden or maple syrup
- Sponge and custard
- Fruit crumbles and custard
- Milk puddings
- Instant whips
- Yogurt and Müllerice

APPENDIX V: FOOD-BASED STANDARDS IN SCHOOLS

The following are food-based standards now in operation in primary, secondary and special schools.

Fruit and vegetables
In all forms (fresh, frozen, canned, dried or juice).

Not less than two portions per day per child, at least one of which should be salad or vegetables, and at least one should be fresh fruit, fruit tinned in juice or fruit salad (fresh or tinned in juice). A fruit-based dessert shall be available at least twice per week.

Meat, fish and other non-dairy sources of protein
Meat (including ham and bacon), fish (fresh, frozen, canned or dried), eggs, nuts, pulses and beans (other than green beans).

A food from this group should be available on a daily basis. Red meat to be available twice a week; fish once a week, and oily fish at least once every three weeks.

Starchy foods
These include all bread (e.g. chapattis), pasta, noodles, rice, potatoes, sweet potatoes, yams, millet and cornmeal.

A food from this group should be available on a daily basis. Fat or oil shall not be used in the cooking process of starchy foods on more than three days in any week. On every day that a fat or oil is used in the cooking process of starchy foods, a starchy food for which fat or oil is not used in the cooking process should also be available. In addition bread should be available on a daily basis.

Deep-fried foods
Meals should not contain more than two deep-fried items in a single week, including products that are deep-fried in the manufacturing process.

Milk and dairy foods
Including milk, cheese, yogurt (including frozen and drinking yogurt), fromage frais and custard.

A food from this group should be available on a daily basis.

Drinks
The only drinks available should be plain water (still or fizzy), milk (skimmed or

semi-skimmed), pure fruit juices, yogurt or milk drinks (with less than 5 per cent added sugar), and drinks made from combinations of any of these (e.g. smoothies), low calorie hot chocolate, tea and coffee. (Artificial sweeteners could be used only in yogurt and milk drinks; or combinations containing yogurt or milk.)

Confectionery and savoury snacks

Confectionery, chocolate and chocolate coated products (excluding cocoa powder used in chocolate cakes, or low calorie hot drinking chocolate) shall not be available throughout the lunch time. The only savoury snacks available should be nuts and seeds with no added salt or sugar.

APPENDIX VI: DIETITIANS IN SPORT AND EXERCISE NUTRITION (DISEN)

Dietitians in Sport and Exercise Nutrition (DISEN) is a specialist group of the British Dietetic Association.

All members of DISEN are professionally qualified dietitians who are state registered.

State registration is issued by the Dietitians Board of the Health Professions Council, and is reviewed and updated annually. All state-registered dietitians must work within the Statement of Conduct issued by the Dietitians Board.

In addition, many members are registered sport and exercise nutritionists, having undertaken further training in the specialist area of sports nutrition, and have a post-graduate qualification in sports dietetics. The register is overseen by the SENr Board that has representatives from each of the three partner organizations, namely The British Dietetic Association, The British Association for Sport and Exercise Sciences and The Nutrition Society. The Board also has a representative from UK Sport and has an independent Chair.

Sports dietitians provide expert advice on all areas of nutrition for sport and exercise. They provide practical help on diet, adapting it to suit individual sports, training programmes and lifestyles.

www.disen.org

References

Chapter 1

1. Department of Health *Dietary Reference Values for Food Energy and Nutrients for the United Kingdom* London: HMSO, 1991. Report on Health and Social Subjects; No. 41.

Chapter 2

1. W. N. Schofield, C. Scholfield, W. P. T. James (1985) Basal metabolic rate – review and prediction *Human Nutrition: Clinical Nutrition*, 39 (suppl.), 1–96.
2. K. Foster-Powell, S. H. A. Holt, J. C. Brand-Miller (2002) 'International table of glycaemic index and glycaemic load values: 2002' *American Journal Clinical Nutrition* 76, 5–56.

Chapter 3

1. W. D. McArdle, F. I. Katch, V. L. Katch (1999) *Sports and Exercise Nutrition* Philadelphia: Lipincott Williams & Wilkins.
2. M. N. Sawka, L. M. Burke, E. R. Eichner, R. J. Maughan, S. J. Montain, N. S. Stachenfeld (2007) 'Position Stand. Exercise and Fluid Replacement' *Medicine and Science in Sports and Exercise*, 39 (2), 377–390.
3. R. J. Maughan, S. M. Shirreffs, J. B. Leiper (2007) 'Errors in the estimation of hydration status from changes in body mass' *Journal of Sports Sciences*, 25 (7), 797–804.
4. R. J. Maughan, J. Griffin (2003) 'Caffeine ingestion and fluid balance: a review' *Journal of Human Nutrition*, 16, 411–420.
5. C. A. Piantadosi (2006) '"Oxygenated" water and athletic performance' *British Journal of Sports Medicine*, 40, 740.

Chapter 4

1. G. M. Duthie (2006) 'A framework for the physical development of élite rugby union players' *International Journal Sports Physiology and Performance*, 1, 2–13.
2. C. Williams, L. Serratosa (2006) 'Nutrition on match day' *Journal of Sports Sciences*, 24 (7), 687–697.
3. B. Lundy, H. O'Connor, F. Pelly, I. Caterson (2006) 'Anthropometric characteristics and competition dietary intakes of professional rugby league players' *International Journal of Sport Nutrition and Exercise Metabolism*, 16, 199–213.

Chapter 5

1. J. A. Hawley, K. D. Tipton, M. L. Millard-Stafford (2006) 'Promoting training adaptations through nutritional interventions' *Journal of Sports Sciences*, 24, 709-721.
2. J. E. Schoffstall, J. D. Branch, B. C. Leutholtz, D. P. Swain (2001) 'Effects of dehydration and rehydration on the one-repetition maximum bench press of weight-trained males' *Journal of Strength and Conditioning Research*, 15 (1), 102–108.

Chapter 6

1. W. J. Kraemer, J. C. Torine, R. Silvestre, D. N. French, N. A. Ratamess, B. A. Spiering, D. L. Hatfield, J. L. Vingren, J. S. Volek (2005) 'Body size and composition of national football league players' *The Journal of Strength and Conditioning Research*, 19 (3), 485–489.
2. T. J. Gabbett (2005) 'Changes in physiological and anthropometric characterics of rugby league players during a competitive season' *Journal of Strength and Conditioning Research* 2005; 19(2): 400–408.
3. B. J. Rolls , E. A. Bell . (1999) 'Intake of fat and carbohydrate: role of energy density' *European Journal of Clinical Nutrition*, 53 S166–S173.
4. R. J. Moffat, S. A. Chelland (2004) 'Carnitine. *Nutritional ergogenic aids*' edited by I. Wolinsky and J. A. Driskell. CRC Press LLC, 61–79.
5. A. Golay, A.-F. Allaz, J. Ybarra, P. Bianchi, S. Saraiva, N. Mensi, R. Gomis, N. de Tonnac (2000) 'Similar weight loss with low energy food combining or balanced diets' *International Journal of Obesity*, 24, 492–496.
6. B. J. Rolls, L. S. Roe, J. S. Meengs, D. E. Wall (2004) 'Increasing the portion size of a sandwich increases energy intake.' *Journal of the American Dietetic Association*; 104 (3), 367–372.
7. W. H. Saris, A. Astrup , A. Prentice, Zunft,

X.Formiguera, W. P. H. G. Verboeket-van de Venne, A. Raben, S. D. Poppitt, S. Johnston, T. H. Vasilaras, G. F. Keogh (2000) 'Randomised controlled trial of changes in dietary carbohydrate/fat ratio and simple vs. complex carbohydrates on bodyweight and blood lipids: the Carmen Study' *International Journal of Obesity*, 24, 1310–1318.

8. Hasler G., Buysse M. D., Klaghofer R., Gamma A., Ajdacic V., Eich D., Rossler W., Angst J. (2004) 'The association between short sleep duration and obesity in young adults: a 13-year prospective study' *Sleep*, 27 (4), 661–666.

Chapter 7

1. J. J. Winnick, M. J. Davis, R. S. Welsh, M. D. Carmichael, D. Martin, A. E. Murphy, J. A. Blackmon (2005) 'Carbohydrate feedings during team sport exercise preserve physical and CNS function' *Medicine and Science in Sports and Exercise*, 37 (2), 306–315.

2. G. R. Cox *et al.* (2002) 'Effect of different protocols of caffeine intake on metabolism and endurance performance' *Journal of Applied Physiology*, 93, 990–999.

3. M. Doherty, P. M. Smith (2004) 'Effects of caffeine ingestion on exercise testing: A meta-analysis' *International Journal of Sport Nutrition and Exercise Metabolism*, 14, 626–646.

4 G. R. Stuart, W. G. Hopkins, C. Cook, S. P. Cairns (2005) 'Multiple effects of caffeine on simulated high-intensity team-sport performance' *Medicine and Science in Sports and Exercise*, 37 (11), 1998–2005.

5. D. M. O'Connor, M. J. Crowe (2003) 'Effects of β-hydroxy-β-methylbutyrate and creatine monohydrate supplementation on the aerobic and anaerobic capacity of highly trained athletes' *Journal of Sports Medicine and Physical Fitness*, 43, 64–68.

Chapter 8

1. Department of Health (DH) *Dietary Reference Values for Food Energy and Nutrients for the United Kingdom* 'Report of the Panel on Dietary Reference Values of the Committee on Medical Aspects of Food Policy.' *Report on Public Health and Social Subjects 41*, London HMSO, 1991.

2. B. R. Stephens, A. S. Cole, A. D. Mahon (2006) 'The influence of biological maturation on fat and carbohydrate metabolism during exercise in males' *International Journal of Sport Nutrition and Exercise Metabolism*, 16, 166–179.

3. B. W. Timmins, O. Bar-Or, M. C. Riddell (2003) Oxidation rate of exogenous carbohydrate during exercise is higher in boys than in men. *Journal of Applied Physiology*, 94 (1), 278–284.

4. N. Boisseau, C. LeCreff, M.Loyens, J. R. Poortmans, (2002) 'Protein intake and nitrogen balance in male non-active adolescents and soccer players' *European Journal of Applied Physiology*, 88, 288–293.

5. Wilk B., Bar-Or O. (1996) 'Effect of drink flavor and NaCl on voluntary drinking and rehydration in boys exercising in the heat' *Journal of Applied Physiology*, 80, 1112–1117.

6. American College of Sports Medicine (2000) 'The physiological and health effects of oral creatine supplementation' *Medicine and Science in Sports and Exercise*, 32, 706–717.

Chapter 9

1. J. H. M. Brooks, C. W. Fuller, S. P. T. Kemp, D. B. Reddin (2005) 'Epidemiology of injuries in English professional rugby union: Part 1 match injuries' *British Journal of Sports Medicine*, 39, 757–766.

2. J. H. M. Brooks, C. W. Fuller, S. P. T. Kemp, D. B. Reddin (2005) 'Epidemiology of injuries in English professional rugby union: Part 2 training injuries' *British Journal of Sports Medicine*, 39, 767–775.

3. J. H. M. Brooks, C. W. Fuller, S. P. T. Kemp, D. B. Reddin (2005) 'A prospective study of injuries and training amongst the England 2003 Rugby World Cup squad' *British Journal of Sports Medicine*, 39, 288–293.

4. T. J. Gabbett (2004) 'Influence of training and match intensity on injuries in rugby league' *Journal Sports Sciences*, 22, 409–417.

5. P. Hespel, B. Op't Eijnde, M. Van Leemputte, B. Urso, P. Greenhaff, V. Lararque (2001) 'Oral creatine supplementation facilitates the rehabilitation of disuse atrophy and alters the expression of muscle myogenic factors in humans' *Journal of Physiology*, 76, 1043–1048

6. R. L. Clancy, M. Gleeson, A. Cox, R. Callister, M. Dorrington, C. D'Este, G. Pang, D. Pyne, P. Fricker, A. Henriksson (2006) 'Reversal in fatigued athletes of a defect in interferon γ secretion after administration of Lactobacillus acidophilus' *British Journal of Sports Medicine*, 40, 351–354.

7. C. Curtis, S. Rees, R. Evans, C. M. Dent, B. Caterson, J. L. Harwood (2004) 'The effects of n-3 polyunsaturated fatty acids on cartilage metabolism in patients with osteoarthritis: the results of a pilot clinical trial. *Proceedings of the third European Federation for the Science and Technology of Lipids*, Edinburgh, 5–8 September, p.216.

8. D. O. Clegg *et al.* (2006) 'Glucosamine, chondroitin sulfate, and the two in combination for painful knee osteoarthritis' *New England Medical Journal of Medicine*, 354, 795–808.

Useful Addresses and Websites

The British Dietetic Association

5th Floor
Charles House
148/9 Great Charles Street Queensway
Birmingham
B3 3HT
www.bda.uk.com

British Nutrition Foundation
High Holborn House
52-54 High Holborn
London
WC1V 6RQ
www.nutrition.org.uk

Dietitians in Sport and Exercise Nutrition
PO Box 176
Stockport
Cheshire
SK7 1XZ
www.disen.org

Food Standards Agency
UK Office
Aviation House
125 Kingsway
London
WC2B 6NH
www.foodstandards.gov.uk
www.eatwell.gov.uk

The Nutrition Society
10 Cambridge Court
210 Shepherds Bush Road
London
W6 7NJ
www.nutritionsociety.org

Sports Council for Northern Ireland
House of Sport
Upper Malone Road
Belfast
BT9 5LA
www.sportni.net

Sports Council for Wales
Sophia Gardens
Cardiff
CF11 9SW
www.sports-council-wales.org.uk

Sport England
3rd Floor
Victoria House
Bloomsbury Square
London
WC1B 4SE
www.sportengland.org

Sportscotland
Caledonia House
South Glye
Edinburgh
EH12 9DQ
www.sportscotland.org.uk

UK Sport
40 Bernard Street
London
WC1N 1ST
www.uksport.gov.uk

USEFUL WEBSITES

American College of Sports Medicine: *www.acsm.org*

Australian Institute of Sport: *www.ais.org.au*

British Association of Sport and Exercise Medicine:
www.basem.co.uk
British Association of Sport and Exercise Sciences:
www.bases.org.uk

Gatorade Sports Science Institute:
www.gssiweb.com

Lucozade Sport Science Academy: *www.thelssa.com*

World Anti-Doping Agency:
www.wada-ama.org

Dietetic Organizations

American Dietetic Association: *www.eatright.org*

Sports, Cardiovascular and Wellness Nutritionists Dietetic Practice Group: *www.scanpg.org*

Dietitians Association of Australia: *www.daa.asn.au*

Sports Dietitians Australia: *www.sportsdietitians.com.au*

Dietitians of Canada: *www.dietitians.ca*

New Zealand Dietetic Association: *www.dietitians.org.nz*

Association for Dietetics in South Africa: *www.adsa.org.za*

RUGBY WEBSITES

International Rugby Board: *www.irb.com*

English Rugby Football Union: *www.rfu.com*

Irish Rugby Football Union: *www.irishrugby.ie*

Scottish Rugby Union: *www.scottishrugby.org*

Welsh Rugby Union: *www.wru.co.uk*

Australian Rugby Union: *www.rugby.com.au*

French Rugby Union: *www.ffr.fr*

Italian Rugby Union: *www.federugby.it*

New Zealand Rugby Football Union: *www.nzrugby.co.nz*

South African Rugby Football Union: *www.sarugby.co.za*

UK Rugby Magazines

Rugby World
England Rugby – the official magazine of the RFU

Index